MW01378130

THE

ART OF DISPENSING

ART OF DISPENSING:

A TREATISE ON

THE METHODS AND PROCESSES INVOLVED IN

COMPOUNDING MEDICAL PRESCRIPTIONS.

THIRD EDITION.

Published at the Offices of

THE CHEMIST AND DRUGGIST,

42 CANNON STREET, LONDON, E.C.

AND NORMANBY CHAMBERS, MELBOURNE.

1888.

PREFACE.

THE treatises on dispensing which formed the literary portions of *The Chemists' and Druggists' Diaries* for 1880 and 1885 attempted, with a large measure of success, to fill a gap in English pharmaceutical literature. Numerous as are the commentaries upon the British Pharmacopœia and the treatises on Galenical pharmacy, there existed no book in our literature which dealt solely with the work of the dispensing counter. For this reason the 1885 treatise on dispensing has been much sought after, especially from the fact that it was a work to which several of the most eminent British pharmacists had contributed, amongst them being Messrs. A. W. Gerrard, W. Gilmour, Thomas Greenish, Joseph Ince, T. Maben, W. Martindale, B. S. Proctor, and others. Continental methods were represented in the volume by extracts from Dr. Hermann Hager's 'Technik der Pharmaceutischen Receptur,' and medical opinion on dispensing matters found an able exponent in Dr. Whitla.

In the present treatise the main features of the 1885 work have been retained, together with the more important of the contributions of the before-named authorities; but, while the most useful parts of that work have been retained, many new features have been introduced; the work as a whole has been rewritten, and the enlarged size of the book shows that it has been greatly extended.

While the treatise retains its character as a compendium for the dispensing counter and as a reference book for the chemist's library, students—medical and pharmaceutical—will, it is hoped, find it of value as a text-book for examinational purposes. Teachers of pharmacy may use it as the basis of their instruction, all the prescriptions given in the work being the actual prescriptions of medical practitioners.

Several of the illustrations are reproductions of drawings from Professor Remington's ' Practice of Pharmacy,' which the Editor of *The Chemist and Druggist* begs to acknowledge. It is also right to add that the work in its present form has been partly written and entirely edited by Mr. Peter MacEwan, F.C.S., pharmaceutical chemist, of the editorial staff of *The Chemist and Druggist.*

THE first edition of this treatise was published on September 18, and was entirely exhausted in three weeks. The present edition is substantially a reprint—no material alteration of the text having been attempted—but the typographical errors of the first edition have been removed.

THE second edition having been disposed of even more rapidly than the first, this reprint is now issued.

42 CANNON STREET, LONDON, E.C.
November, 1888.

CONTENTS.

vii · *CONTENTS*

THE
ART OF DISPENSING.

—◦—

GENERAL SUGGESTIONS.

The Dispenser must cultivate habits of order and cleanliness. Dirtiness and untidiness in dress in the dispenser must give the public an unpleasant impression. Such practices as pressing corks with the teeth, holding powder-envelopes in the mouth, shaking up mixtures with the finger over the mouth of the bottle, breathing on pills to be silvered should be avoided. Decent and becoming manners are essential. Scolding the apprentice and joking with his fellow-assistants are equally out of place, and should be carefully avoided in the pharmacy at all times. Dispensing is the most responsible part of the pharmacist's duties, and is considered to be so by doctors and patients alike; the closest attention and the most scrupulous care should, therefore, be manifested at the dispensing counter.

Quality of Drugs.—The medicines employed in the preparation of prescriptions should be of the finest quality procurable for money, and officinal or other preparations made from them should be prepared in strict accordance with recognised methods. Second qualities of some goods may be necessary for

B

certain purposes in other sales, but the pharmacist should not for a single moment permit the entrance of a thought about second qualities in the dispensing department. Differences will occur in medicines prepared at different establishments, but always at least retain the satisfaction of knowing that these cannot result from the use of inferior drugs in *your* pharmacy. Let the question of profit gained from the dispensing of prescriptions be a secondary one. That will take care of itself. Dispense medicine with the feeling that an artist has in his work, and so will you make an art of your work. Ensure by occasional testing that preparations which are liable to deteriorate are of proper strength ; this applies particularly to such as acid. hydrocyanic. dil. and spt. æther. nitrosi. Although you pay the best price for your drugs, do not let that prevent you submitting them to examination before placing them in stock.

Style in Externals.—The pharmacist, however, may lose all the pecuniary benefit of his conscientiousness if, after using the most costly drugs, he should be wanting in neatness or style in sending them out. The dispenser who economises on his drugs is a rogue, but he who economises on his bottles, corks, pill-boxes, or paper is a fool. Customers can only judge by the externals, and generally they would be right in concluding that a man who sends out his drugs in a low-class bottle with a brittle cork may have used drugs of equally low quality. Evidence of slovenliness on the outside of a packet does not encourage faith as to the care with which the contents have been combined. Some taste may be shown in labels as well as in the boxes, bottles, &c., upon which they are placed. Let the direction to the patient and not your own name and address be the most prominent part of the label. Have a nice neat label for the dispensing department, with as little beyond your name, qualification, and address as you can help.

On this subject Professor Remington remarks that 'neatness, distinctness, and simplicity are cardinal principles in designing labels, and the reputation of many establishments is frequently judged from the character of the outward signs of neatness and care. For this reason particular attention should be paid to prescription-labels, not only to have the printed address plain, clear, and neat, but to have the handwriting to correspond. In these important particulars patients are exceedingly apt to form an estimate of the qualifications of the compounder of a prescription from the style of his penmanship, reasoning that, if he is careful, clean, and neat in the one particular of which they are competent to judge—*i.e.* the handwriting on the label—the compounder must exercise similar qualifications in the more vital operations involved in compounding and dispensing, for upon the technicalities of the latter they cannot hope to pass judgment.'

In a competition in *The Chemist and Druggist* we had an extensive variety of labels and specimens of handwriting, and from these we give a selection. The first label is that to which the prize was awarded for distinctness.

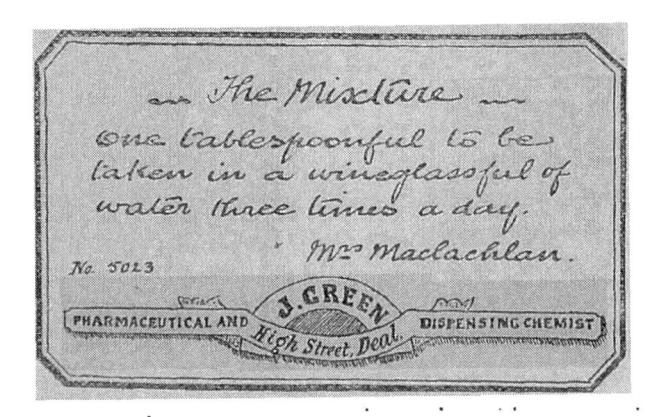

This label exhibits with fair accuracy what a writer has put down as a cardinal principle in writing directions upon a label— viz. to balance the matter so that its parts may form a sym-·metrical arrangement. All the lines must begin and terminate at the same distance from the margin. If we write 'The Mixture,' or 'The Powders,' we must take care that it is exactly in the centre. The appearance of a label is greatly marred by having it nearer to one side than the other. We

must also be careful to manage the adjustment of the matter
so that it may fill the label pretty well.   To have a label with
two lines of writing at the top and three lines unoccupied at the
bottom is to sacrifice its proportion.   It is in this connection
that a middling writer who has an eye for proportion in form
may surpass a good writer in execution of a label.   The free
and easy writer too often trusts so much to the excellence of
his work that he altogether neglects the just apportionment of
its parts.

It is desirable to have more than one kind of dispensing
label, so that if more than one internal remedy is dispensed
for a patient, or two or more patients in one family, there may
be distinctiveness in the externals.   Upright labels such as the
following are very serviceable in this respect.   These, we may
say, are only half-size reproductions :—

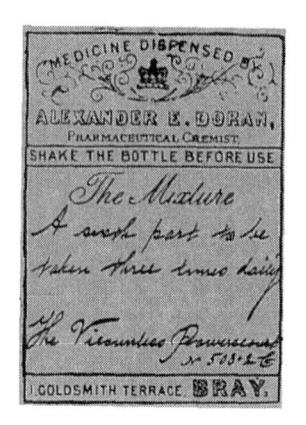 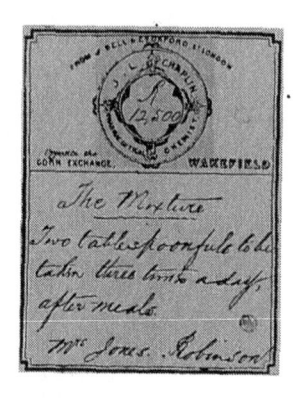

It is a good thing also to have different shaped bottles, such
as dispensing 'flats,' ovals, and squares.   Instead of having the
words 'Mixture,' 'Lotion,' &c., printed on the label it has been
suggested to have indiarubber stamps for these words.   This
is an economical and on the whole a serviceable plan to those
who cannot afford a variety of labels.   In round labels there is
little room for variety, but in this case it is all the more import-.
ant, owing to the small space for directions, to have little room
wasted on the name and address.   We give two specimens

of round labels, one of which shows the utility of the type-writer :—

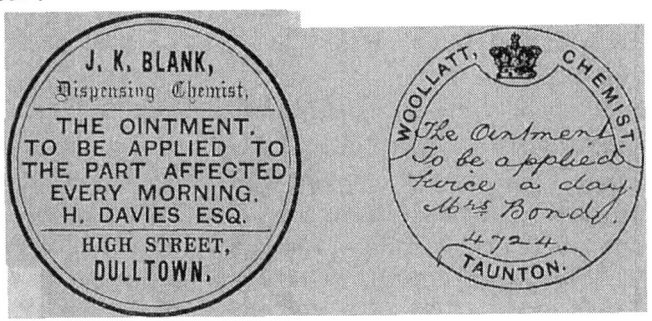

The foregoing examples show several styles of handwriting. The ability to write neatly is a very important requisite for the dispenser. Bad penmanship is too easily accepted as a sort of natural defect, and a good many people even pride themselves on it. Some perseverance, however, is all that is necessary to make a bad writer into a good one, and the youth who will not take the trouble to cultivate that first branch of his art had better abandon any thought of fitting himself to become a dispenser of medicines.

Labels should always be neatly trimmed by carefully cutting off with a pair of scissors the surplus paper at the margin. Many pharmacists omit to do this, although it adds greatly to the 'finish' and elegant appearance.

The rare, but not unknown, practice of placing a fresh label over an old one to save the trouble of removing it should on no account be permitted. Apart from the slovenliness, such a habit may produce mistakes from the accidental removal of the top label and exposure of another unlike in nature or dose. It .is often advisable to re-label. The old label can be quickly removed by damping with water and holding it over the gas flame or before the fire for a few seconds. This softens the mucilage, and the label may be removed with ease.

'**Poison**,' 'Shake the bottle,' and other adventitious labels are best placed at the shoulder of the bottle. If placed at the foot, the hand holding the bottle may cover them, or a hurried person may overlook them.   At the shoulder they will be read first.   Moreover, it frequently happens that the patient will only tear off the upper part of the wrapper ; hence a label at the bottom of the bottle in this case would be of no avail, because not seen.

Another plan which is equally efficient, and neater, is to have 'Poison' and 'Shake the bottle' printed on the labels. One series of lotion labels may be had with 'Poison,' at the top, and another series without.   In the same way, mixture labels may be had of two series—one with a plain 'The Mixture,' and the other with 'Shake the bottle before using' printed immediately below 'The Mixture,' or at the bottom of the blank space.   Orange-coloured paper is very commonly used for poison labels, and is undoubtedly very distinctive ; but it has one disadvantage.   When used for liniments of an oily nature, the labels are apt to get stained, and the stains almost completely hide the printing and writing.

Capping Bottles.—In capping bottles with leather it is a good plan to soak for a short time in lime water (which bleaches it), or even in plain water.   Crimson paper is generally used for capping (in the manner shown in the accompanying figure), but it is now largely giving way to Hunt's pleated caps.   If you tie on a cap with string, form a loop knot, so that string and cap may be removed together.

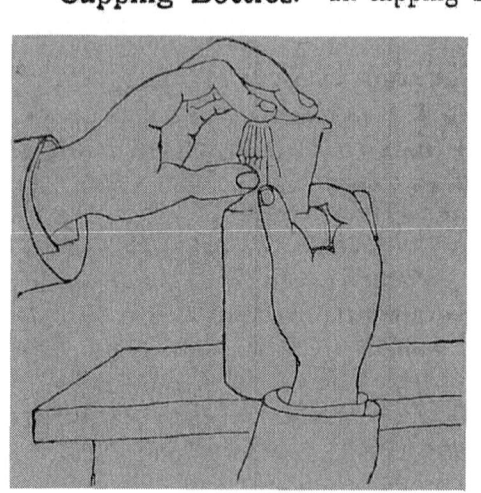

HOW TO MAKE A PLEATED PAPER CAP EXTEMPORANEOUSLY.

One thing at a time.—Never have two prescriptions

going at once. Of course, if there is an infusion to make, you will set that on—set the jar on one side, marking on a piece of paper what it is, and hold that label between the cover and the jar. You can then go on with another prescription. But, having finished one, clear up all mess, and put away bottles, measures, and mortars, before beginning anything else. Indeed, bottles, measures, and mortars should be replaced directly after being used, and should on no account be allowed to accumulate on the counter.

Checking.—It is desirable that one person should copy the prescription, write the labels and dispense the medicine. The copying should always precede the dispensing, and the dispenser will then have acquired a general acquaintance with the prescription. If the staff is large enough, it is a very good plan for a second person to examine the medicine, compare the labels with the prescription, and finish off. In any case, the dispenser should never let his medicine leave him without making a final reading of the prescription, concentrating all his attention on it, and considering whether he has exactly followed the instructions. He may, for example, have used citrate of iron when citrate of iron and quinine was ordered, and he would hardly fail to recognise this oversight if he devoted a few final moments to the work of supervision. He should, last of all, give a final reading to his copy, carefully noting the quantities as well as the substances.

Precautions.—In large dispensing businesses, where it may happen that medicines are handed to customers out of a considerable number of packages, Dr. Hager recommends the employment of duplicate numbers. A certain figure is given to the person ordering the medicine, and a corresponding number is attached to the prescription itself, so as to guard against the possible occasional delivery of the wrong medicine. The plan would have an air of absurdity in any but the chief businesses, but it would have a good effect where it could be reasonably employed.

Another suggestion is that on the back of the label, or at

the bottom of the box, shall be printed a form, something like this :—

Prescription received . . . . . 3.10 P.M.
Medicine ready . . . . . . 3.30 ,,
Delivered to messenger . . . . . 4 ,,

The advantage of this is shown by citing the case of a messenger who, having wasted several hours in the town and taken the medicine home after the patient had died, pretended that he was detained by the pharmacist, but whose false statement was refuted by a label like the above.

A more important detail even than this, and one which is now very common in larger dispensing establishments, is to attach a small label to each box, bottle, or pot, &c., initialed by the dispenser, and also by the checker, previous to wrapping it up and sending it out. Thus :—

Dispensed by A. B.
Checked by C. D.

The advantages of this plan are obvious. There is the probability of detecting any serious blunder, while if it is checked by a superior it is calculated to act as a deterrent to slurring the dispensing in any way.

Whether these precautions are used or not, a prescription-register should certainly be kept. Here we reproduce the ruling of the register of one of the principal dispensing establishments in the kingdom, but which is also in use in small establishments where only two apprentices and no assistants are kept. The advantages which are claimed for this are : (1) It shows the amount of dispensing done in a day, week, month, or year ; (2) the nature of the medicine dispensed ; (3) the hour when dispensed (this is a check upon delivery should the messenger have put off time) ; and (4) the names of the dispenser and checker. We note the width of each column :—

Date	Name	Address	Medicine	Number	Hour	Dispensed by	Checked by
Feb. 5	Betsy Jones	Glad- stone Place	6 oz. mixture	42,356	10.50	A. B.	C. D.
½ in.	1¾ in.	1⅞ in.	1 in.	1 in.	¾ in.	¾ in.	¾ in.

A great deal is, however, to be said against all methods if you employ them simply in order to impress upon patients how careful you are. Remember that every effort should be made to attain *absolute* correctness in dispensing and promptitude in delivery of medicines ; perfect satisfaction is thus guaranteed, and complaints will be extremely rare. If the prescription-register has to be often referred to for the purpose of detecting culprits, that only proves that it has failed in its chief function. Mistakes should *never* be allowed to occur, and the most certain indication of accurate dispensing and careful checking is that the register never requires to be reopened. Good general supervision by the principal for the time being should never be neglected.

GIVING COPIES OF PRESCRIPTIONS.

The following is a brief summary of a series of letters published in the April number of *The Chemist and Druggist*, 1884, on the question, Has a customer a right to demand a copy of a prescription from a pharmacist?

'Midland Chemist' had in his books a copy of a prescription entered in 1860. The original owner had been dead three years, and a member of his family asked for a copy to circulate and do good in a neighbourhood ten or twelve miles away.

Mr. Eve (of Messrs. Allen and Hanburys) says the copies of prescriptions are only made for a definite legal purpose and confer no right upon the owner. When copies have become valuable property no reasonable customer would persist in asking for them.

Mr. F. Andrews (London) thinks it would be perfectly right to decline to give a copy.

Mr. Daniel Frazer holds that the patient is the owner of the prescription, not the prescriber or the pharmacist. As to the dispenser giving copies of prescriptions entered in his books, each man must judge for himself. The pharmacist should never hesitate to give a copy when requested by the original owner.

Mr. Thomas Greenish (London): Prescriptions are copied at the expense of the pharmacist, who has a sole right to the copies, the original prescription only being the property of the patient for whom it was written. To give a copy is a matter of courtesy.

Mr. William Gilmour (Edinburgh): Entering a prescription into a prescription-book in no way invests the chemist with any proprietary right in it. He would not take the responsibility of trading in any prescription or of giving a copy of it to any but the original holder, or at his request.

Mr. Joseph Ince (London): It is probably not legal that a particular recipe should be retained by the pharmacist. But the book of manuscript copied prescriptions is the property of the dispenser—part of his stock—and can be bought or sold. No one but the original owner has even the claim of courtesy to assert in desiring a copy.

Mr. William Martindale (London): The only persons who can show a title of claim to a copy of a prescription copied in a chemist's prescription-book (and these only by favour) are the prescriber and the patient. If both prescriber and patient are dead, the copy is ethically the chemist's *in toto*. Your copy is no longer a prescription.

Mr. R. Reynolds (Leeds): Your correspondent may refuse to give a copy of the prescription alluded to without anyone having a remedy at law against him. To give away valuable parts of his prescription-books, bought as part of the goodwill, would be damaging his future and drawing upon his capital.

Mr. G. F. Schacht (Bristol) considers the original prescription itself to be the property of the patient, and the copy of that prescription in the chemist's book to be the property of the chemist. The chemist could scarcely refuse to give a copy to the patient; but when the latter dies the chemist's one and only obligation ceases, and it rests entirely upon his judgment and his courtesy whether he shall part with a copy to anyone.

Dr. Charles Symes (Liverpool): As a matter of courtesy it is well to give a copy of a prescription when it is required for a legitimate purpose, always holding the right to refuse it if required for the furtherance of quackery or for use to the direct prejudice of the pharmacist possessing it.

The late Mr. William Southall (Birmingham): The copy of a prescription is an assistance to memory, in which no one can claim any right or property but the copyist. The original holder of the prescription has no ownership in the copy. On the other hand, a chemist has no right to dispense any prescription of which he may possess a copy, as being Mr. So-and-so's, without the owner's permission.

Our Legal Contributor : The chemist does not acquire the right to use the property of a patient (whose prescription he has copied) as part of his stock-in-trade, for the purpose of making money thereby. The customer has no right to demand a copy from the prescription-book on the ground that he has lost the original prescription. If a customer allows the chemist to use the medicine for various purposes and to take the profit arising from the sale thereof, and this continues for a long course of years, in the absence of any proof to the contrary it would be assumed that the owner had given the chemist a general right to make up the medicine for his own profit.

INCE'S DISPENSING APHORISMS.

Read through a prescription, rapidly and in a manner suggesting no suspicion of doubt. Write directions invariably before dispensing. Avoid thus the use of blotting-paper : a good dispenser uses almost none. If a mixture contains readily soluble ingredients, never use a mortar. Avoid effecting solution by heat, for fear of recrystallisation. With syrups and also ingredients not water, arrange in dispensing to rinse out the measure and leave it clean. A skilled dispenser shows very little traces of his work. Carefully clean and put away weights and scales after each operation. Hold the scales firmly by the left hand ; never lift them high above the counter ; and judge of the weight as much by the indicator as by the position of the scale. Select glass pans for scales—preferably of heavy make— and discard flimsy brass material, which corrodes speedily, and becomes inaccurate. Learn to judge of the quantity to be weighed with tolerable accuracy : train the eye as well as the hand. If in doubt, always begin with that of which you have no doubt. Be rapid in manipulation. Finish wrapping, tying, or sealing quickly. Slow dispensing is bad dispensing, and arises either from deficient practice or want of knowledge. Never, when in a shadow of doubt, hesitate to ask advice from a fear of compromising your own dignity.

LEEDS & WEST-RIDING

MEDICO-CHIRURGICAL SOCIETY

WEIGHTS AND MEASURES.

Signs.—In 1877 Dr. Redwood gave an authoritative and reasonable explanation of what is to be understood by the various signs for weights and measures. He pointed out that the British Pharmacopœia adopts the avoirdupois weights, and the signs employed—lb., oz., gr.—apply to the weights of this system. The other signs—℈, ʒ, ℥, ℔—however, mean what they always meant—namely, the scruple, drachm, ounce, and pound of the apothecaries' system. The only difficulties can occur in the ounce and pound. Strictly speaking, therefore, it should be understood that ℥ means an apothecaries' or troy ounce of 480 grains, while 'oz.' means an avoirdupois ounce of $437\frac{1}{2}$ grains. So ℔ is the troy pound of 12 troy ounces, and lb. is the avoirdupois pound of 16 avoirdupois ounces. The terms C and O, which formerly designated the wine gallon and pint, are now used in the Pharmacopœia to represent the imperial gallon and pint. This must necessarily be the case, because no other fluid measures are now legal in trade transactions. In weights it is necessary to have a distinction of signs, because the law expressly permits the use of apothecaries' weight in the sale of drugs.

The Pharmacopœia of 1885 introduced for the first time the **fluid grain** in the formulæ for certain preparations, especially some *liquores*. This measure is the bulk of 1 grain of water at the normal conditions, and it was officialised in order to bring potent preparations more into conformity with Continental custom. For example, liquor arsenicalis now contains 1 grain of arsenious acid in 100 fluid grains (or 110 minims), whereas formerly it contained 1 grain in 120 minims. The fluid grain is not, however, recognised in dispensing.

The weights and measures in use in the United States are different from the British. The pint is only 16 ounces, and the ounce is equivalent to 455·7 grains. As in Great Britain, the fluid ounce is divided into 480 minims. The British minim is equal to 0·9114 grain, whereas the American is 0·9285 grain. This difference should be noted in dispensing American prescriptions.

The Metric System is exclusively employed on the Continent, and both liquids and solids are weighed. To convert the weights into English grains it is generally sufficient to multiply the number of grammes by 15. The following are closely approximate values of the more common terms: One gramme = $15\frac{2}{8}$ grains; 1 grain = 6 centigrammes; 1 kilogramme = 2 lb. 3 oz. (av.); 1 lb. (av.) = 456 grammes; 1 oz. avoirdupois = $28\frac{1}{2}$ grammes; 1 cubic centimetre = $16\frac{1}{4}$ minims. It is fairly accurate to reckon that 30 grammes of water or similar liquids are equal to 1 fluid ounce; but it is always preferable to weigh all the ingredients as would be done on the Continent. The tare of the bottle is taken with a quantity of small shot contained in a chip box.

In mixing fluids for a mixture, the rule is, with some exceptions, to put the smallest quantity ordered in the bottle first, then the next largest quantity, and so on. The reason is that the delicacy of the scales diminishes with the increased weight, and as the medicines ordered in small quantities are generally the most powerful, they need to be dispensed with the greatest degree of accuracy. When so many drops of a fluid are ordered it is usual to put the drops in first, so that if a few drops too many fall they can be returned. Fluids up to 1 gramme are generally dropped, and it is reckoned that of the fatty and specifically heavy ethereal oils and of tinctures 20 drops = 1 gramme; of the other ethereal oils, chloroform, acetic ether and spirits of ether, and aqueous fluids, 25 drops = 1 gramme; of ether, 50 drops = 1 gramme. This calculation may not be quite accurate, but it accords with the Prussian medicinal tariff, and is what is understood by the prescribing physician.

The rule thus laid down by Dr. Hager brings out prominently the superiority of the English system of measuring. It has its application, however, to our custom to some extent, the exceptions being where a following of the rule would give a result not desired. The smaller quantities and thinner fluids should

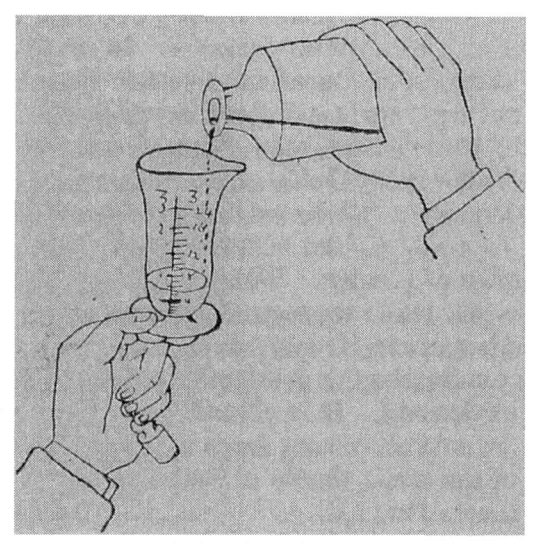

HOW TO MEASURE.

Grasp the measure with the thumb and forefinger of the left hand, the finger being under the measure so as to keep it level. The other fingers thus remain free to grasp the bottle-stopper.

invariably be measured first, or, failing this, measured with a fresh measure-glass. To measure, for example, 1 drachm of hydrocyanic acid after measuring ½ oz. or 1 oz. of glycerine or syrup of squill is clearly to court error. Equally incorrect would it be to start with a 4 oz. measure-glass, however correctly graduated or however suitable for measuring the other ingredients of a prescription, to measure any small quantity of a powerful remedy, such as hydrocyanic acid.

It is much the best plan to make it the practice to use a

separate measure for all potent preparations, such as arsenical solutions, solution of strychnine, hydrocyanic acid and the like, and, if the nature of the mixture permit it, measure such preparations last—that is, after the mixture is made up with water or other diluent, leaving room for the potent preparation.

Carelessness in weighing or measuring is not to be tolerated. There should be if possible, and there generally is in large establishments, a balance for weighing small quantities of alkaloids and other strong remedies. In no case should guesswork exist at the dispensing counter. In mixtures or solutions generally there is little fear that such a course should be adopted; but we have seen doses of powdered opium guessed at by the palette-knife, and so dispensed. We have seen more than once a definite weighed quantity of a compound powder subsequently divided without weighing into the prescribed number of powders. Without assuming that such is a customary practice in some establishments, and recognised as being fairly accurate, its existence is a sufficient justification for strongly condemning this or any other methods which favour dangerous carelessness. It is generally safe to give minims when *guttæ* are ordered, because drops vary in size according to the nature of the liquid, the lip of the bottle, the quantity in the bottle, temperature, &c.

Thus, chloroform dropped from an ordinary phial will give 150 to 300 drops for a fluid drachm. But it is convenient to have the number of drops which equal a drachm marked upon the bottles containing some of the fluids commonly prescribed in small quantities. In some cases it is desirable to weigh rather than measure a liquid—for example, in the case of a dozen minims of croton oil ordered for pills. Here it is practically impossible to get 12 minims of the oil out of a measure once it is in, but it may be weighed on the glass scale-pan, either upon some inert powder, such as soap, previously weighed, or some of the powder may be mixed up with it on the scale-pan and the whole afterwards carefully scraped off. Due allowance has of course to be made for the fact that croton oil is lighter than water, and that a minim of water weighs less than one grain. The average specific gravity of croton oil is ·950, and the weight of a minim of water is ·9114, so that ·950 × ·9114 × 12 = 10·42 (say 10½ grains), the weight of 12 minims of croton oil.

Fractions of a grain are frequently ordered, for example 20 pills each containing $\frac{1}{24}$ grain of strychnine. In this case weigh one grain of alkaloid and triturate it with 11 grains of sugar of milk (which thoroughly divides it), and take 10 grains of the mixture for the 20 pills. A difficulty sometimes is found when fractions of minims are ordered; for example, two pills are ordered each to contain ɱ ⅛ of croton oil and ɱ ¼ of peppermint oil. The best plan in this case is to rub up 1 drop of croton oil and 2 drops of peppermint oil with 10 grains of soap, and take a fourth part of the mixture for the pills.

PRESCRIBERS AND DISPENSERS.

Ambiguous Nomenclature.—More attention by prescribers to the possibilities of *ambiguous nomenclature* would be a great boon to pharmacists. For preparations mentioned in the British Pharmacopœia the name there found should be used, and in ordering those not included in the B.P. the initials of the Pharmacopœia, or the name of the standard work in which the formula may be found, should be appended. No rule can be laid down for the dispenser, except that he should be guided by the date of the prescription. Suppose the following prescription is presented :—

> Tinct. cinchonæ . . . . . . ʒij.
> Sig. ʒi. ter die.
> June 6, 1884.   F. M. H.

The only official simple tincture existing when that prescription was written was *tinctura cinchonæ flavæ.* Now that tincture has been expunged from the Pharmacopœia and a tincture of the red bark has taken its place, but there is no law which compels the dispenser to give the latter tincture in such an instance as the above. The patient has used the old tincture and may prefer it. There are other instances, such as the cases of the liquors which have been slightly altered in strength. Here the dispenser may use the new preparations, because there has been what may be called no material alteration. The following mixture is a very good example of a case in which the substitution of an altered preparation for an old one gives quite a different result :—

Liq. bismuthi et ammon. cit. . . . . . ♏ xx
Liq. magnesiæ bicarb. . . . . . ʒij.
Aquæ . . . . ad ʒss.

Pro dosi. Mitte ʒviii.

Jan. 10, 1885.

The old liquor bismuthi gives a clear mixture ; the new, from its want of excess of ammonium citrate, forms a mixture with a copious precipitate of bismuth.

Dr. Whitla says that the dispenser will often be at a loss to understand the meaning of the prescriber when he orders some preparations out of their official names, and he then must have a consultation, or fall back upon the experience of himself or others. He gives the following examples : When 'magnes. calc.' is ordered, magnesia B.P. should be used ; when 'magnes. carb.' the heavy preparation is usually intended ; when 'bismuth' or 'bismuth alb.' is prescribed, the subnitrate is the preparation generally in the mind of the physician ; when 'aqua menth.' is ordered, aq. menth. pip. should not be used, but aq. menth. sativ. is the intention of the prescriber.

This is a good example of the difference of opinion amongst authorities. In some parts of the country *aq. menthæ virid.* is, no doubt, always dispensed for 'aq. menthæ,' but this custom is not general. Aq. menth. virid. is seldom ordered, but aq. menth. pip. is in daily demand, and is used officially as a flavouring agent. For these reasons it is advisable to use aq. menth. pip. when 'aq. menth.' is ordered, unless the dispenser knows the intention of the prescriber to be the contrary.

Dr. Whitla's remarks regarding magnesia recall a comment which we made in the previous edition. It was then said that 'some apparent difficulties can be settled by reference to the Pharmacopœia—*e.g. Magnesia*, prescribed as such, means the mag. calc. pond. according to the B.P. The light variety is expressly designated *magnesia levis*. This no longer strictly applies, for the term 'magnesia' has been changed to 'magnesia ponderosa,' and 'ponderosa' has also been added to magnesia carbonas. Light carbonate of magnesia is so seldom used, unless in the special cases of inhalation—*e.g.* vapor pini sylvestris—that there should be no hesitation in giving the heavy carbonate when 'magnes. carb.' is ordered. Regarding calcined magnesia, however, the dispenser may well pause and consider questions of bulk, date, &c., before he decides whether he will use the heavy or light.

Amongst other ambiguities of nomenclature, the following are worth notice :—

Acid. nitro-hydrochlor., prescribed without the addition of the qualifying term ' dil.,' is an instance of careless prescribing, but it can hardly occasion a doubt, as the strong compound acid is not official. The *acid. nitro-muriat.* of the Dublin Pharmacopœia is still regularly prescribed by some of the older race of medical men, and a question *might* arise whether this was not intended. Usually, however, this is written in the old style, *acid. nit.-mur.*

Aloes.—The question as to whether Barbadoes or Socotrine aloes should be used when ' aloes ' only occurs in a prescription is one which formerly presented no difficulty, for Socotrine aloes was most commonly employed, Barbadoes aloes being more used for veterinary purposes. Now, however, Socotrine aloes is somewhat variable in quality, while good liver, so-called Barbadoes aloes is effective and thoroughly reliable. This fact should weigh in deciding.

Æther. chlor. is a fruitful source of doubt. It is very general always to dispense the official spirit of chloroform when this is ordered. The only thing against this is that the old chloric ether is a distilled preparation, and is soluble in water. On the whole it is advisable to follow the advice of Squire and others, and use spt. chloroformi unless you know that the distilled preparation is intended : in that case use ' Duncan's.'

When *Ferri cit.* is ordered it is usual to dispense ferri ammon. cit., which is the only official preparation corresponding to the title ; but if a mineral acid be contained in the mixture the simple citrate of iron should be used.

Hyd. chlor. may mean subchloride of mercury, corrosive sublimate, or hydrate of chloral, and mistakes have happened in consequence of this wholly unnecessary abbreviation of terms.

But there is little excuse for a mistake if the dispenser thinks of what he is about. Corrosive sublimate is never given with a purgative or as a sleeping draught, and the whole danger really lies in corrosive sublimate. Reflect before you dispense.

Liq. cinchonæ.—Should Battley's preparation or the pharmacopœial liquid extract be supplied for this? The reply to this is that since the introduction of a formula for liquid extract of cinchona into the Pharmacopœia liq. cinchonæ and ext. cinchon. liq. are synonymous, and when liq. cinchonæ is prescribed without 'Battley's' the dispenser should use the official preparation.

For *liquor ergotæ* give extract. ergotæ liquidum. There need be no hesitation about the matter in these cases : all that you have to consider is that *liquor* is a commonly accepted synonym of *extractum liquidum*, and adherence to the British Pharmacopœia is, in the circumstances, the safest rule for the dispenser to follow.

Liq. morphinæ is very often written in a prescription, and the dispenser will follow the majority in giving liquor morphinæ hydrochlor. There occur exceptions, however ; for instance, a frequent prescription is—

> Liq. plumb. subacet.
>   ,, morphinæ .   .   .   .   .   . a. a. p. æ.

In this case use liq. morph. acet. to avoid precipitation of plumbic chloride. Some physicians use only the acetate of morphine, but such prescribers are generally very particular in specifying what they want.

Liquor taraxaci.—The difficulty regarding the use of the word 'liquor' has recently come up in a new form regarding *liquor taraxaci.* The question was put to us, 'What should be dispensed for this, the *succus* or the liquid extract?' and our reply was to the effect that if the prescription was written *before* the publication of the B.P. 1885, the succus should be dispensed ; but if *after*, the liquid extract. This accords with the rule regarding other liquors. But the answer did not pass unchallenged. One correspondent contested it, thus :—

'The logic of your inference is no doubt correct, but

practice negatives it. "Liq. tarax." has long been synonymous with "succ. tarax." Some wholesale houses used to send out the prescription labelled "Liq. Tarax. (Succ.)." I believe most West-end houses (for whose custom, though, I claim no special merit) would not hesitate to use succ. tarax. B.P. when liq. tarax. is prescribed.'

When, as sometimes happens, *tinct. card.* is prescribed, the dispenser must use his discretion whether a simple tincture or the usual compound tincture is required. In such a case, if the prescription has been previously dispensed, it is best to explain the doubt to the customer, showing him that, though the appearance would differ, the medicinal importance of the difference was but trifling. So also in such cases as tinct. gentianæ, tinct. guaiaci, &c. Generally speaking, it is correct to assume that the prescriber is quite familiar with the British Pharmacopœia, and the dispenser is at all events legally safe in such an assumption.

Questions of Measurement.—The dispenser frequently meets with prescriptions in which it is doubtful what size of mixture the prescriber intends. The following is a good example :—

> Ammonii bromidi . . . . . . ℈iv.
> Syr. chloral hydratis . . . . . ℥i.
> Infusi gentianæ comp. . . . . . ℥vi.
> M. fiat mistura. ℥i. hora somni sumend.

Should this be dispensed as written, as a ℥vi. mixture or as an ℥viii. ? If the dispenser cannot communicate with the prescriber, and has no means of knowing what his intentions in the matter are, the correct plan is to dispense the prescription as written. At the same time, this course would be considered pedantic by many pharmacists, because it is apparent that by making an ℥viii. mixture, a half-drachm dose of ammonium bromide and a drachm dose of syrup of chloral would be contained in each ounce ; and these are most likely intended. One pharmacist who holds this opinion remarks : 'There are cases (and this is one of them) where the dispenser must use his own discretion, and be guided by experience, in trying to find out the intentions of the prescriber, and to do this he must go beyond the bare written instructions. If he does this with tact and to the best of his ability, he will ensure the confidence of the practitioner and his patient, and avoid any need for explanation.'

Always keep in mind that no alteration should be made in a physician's prescription unless that alteration has the prescriber's sanction. Do not of course kill a patient for the sake of a rule. If you make any alteration it should be marked on the prescription, for the guidance of other dispensers.

Familiarity with the prescriptions of a physician obviates difficulties such as that under notice. For example, one physician almost invariably writes his prescription for a mixture thus :—

Potass. bicarb.	ʒij.
Tinct. nuc. vomic.	ʒij.
Syr. aurant.	ʒj.
Inf. quassiæ	℥viij

Ft. mist.

The literal construction of this prescription is to make a ℥ixss. mixture, but the actual intention of the prescriber is known to be only an ℥viii. mixture. In all such cases the dispenser should note the prescription, so that if it strays into the hands of other pharmacists not familiar with the peculiarities of the writer they may not deviate from the original interpretation. This may be done alongside the ℥viii., thus 'ad ℥viii.,' or inside the date stamp.

The Graduation of Medicine Bottles which are to contain mixtures to be taken in parts is a matter which may be considered here. Bottles, being unequal in bore, contain as a rule more near the shoulder than at the base ; and, in consequence, the graduations of spaces do not accurately represent equal divisions of the fluid contents. This does not in ordinary mixtures make much practical difference in the intentions of the prescriber, but may do so in those containing active ingredients, and it is important to ensure accuracy. To show the difference in dosage which results through different methods of graduating, we give an illustration of part of a stock printed slip for a 6 oz. bottle, of which each division represents two tablespoonfuls, the dotted lines at the left representing the bottle graduations which are formed in the mould. This shows conclusively that one, at least, of the methods must be wrong, and very probably both are.

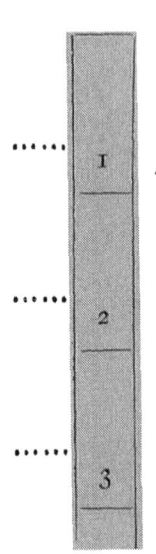

The proper plan is to graduate the bottle by hand. Paste a slip of paper upon the side or back of the bottle, and measure into the bottle the successive parts, indicated by the prescription, marking each part with a short stroke of the pen or pencil, afterwards making a bolder mark when the bottle has been emptied. A small stock of such marked bottles may be kept. Printed slips and moulded graduations have nothing to do with accuracy; they are conveniences. Of course common sense says one may use these conveniences for simple remedies; but where will the line be drawn?

Alteration of Prescriptions.—The question has been put : To what extent is the dispenser justified in effecting the solution or suspension of an ingredient in a mixture which, though prescribed in an insoluble state, is yet to be given in accurately divided doses? The following prescription may be taken as an example :—

Bismuthi subnitratis.	. . . . .	℈ij.
Magnesiæ ponderosæ	. . . . .	℈i.
Tincturæ gentianæ comp. .	. . . .	ʒi.
Aquæ . . .	. . .	ad ℥viii.

Fiat mistura.

Obviously the patient cannot measure out fixed portions of this mixture containing equal doses of bismuth, and the dispenser would do him (or her) a good turn by adding a viscous ingredient to suspend it. Preference should be given to tragacanth mucilage, because it is not only more viscous than acacia mucilage, but contains relatively a much smaller proportion of solid matter. It is noteworthy, however, that if either mucilage is added to bismuth subnitrate, when no other powder is prescribed along with it, the two seem to combine in some way to form a glutinous, indiffusible mass at the bottom of the bottle. Compound tragacanth powder does not have this objection.

Another case may be cited. Is the substitution of liq. arsenici hydrochlor. justifiable in the following prescription ?—

Liq. arsenicalis (Fowler's) .   .   .   .   .   . ℥j.
Liq. hydrarg. perchlor.   .   .   .   .   . ℥j.
Aquæ   .   .   .   .   .   . ad ℥iv.

M. ft. mist. ʒij. t. d. s.

Liquor arsenicalis precipitates the mercury, and there is a possibility of the patient getting the whole of it in the last dose.

An analogous result is shown in mixtures of liq. arsenicalis and liq. strychninæ in certain proportions, the alkaloid being in this case precipitated. In both these cases the acid solution should, preferably, be used, a little compound tincture of lavender being added.

Careless Prescribers.—It would save the pharmacist a great deal of anxiety if prescribers would take the trouble to initial unusual doses, for many instances occur where it is impossible for the dispenser to know whether the dose is safe or not; for instance, the official dose of potassium iodide is 2 to 10 grains, yet 20 grains is a frequent dose, and even 1 or 2 drachms twice or three times a day, while some patients experience very unpleasant effects from a single dose of 2 grains. Again, the official dose of ext. ergotæ liq. is 10 to 30 minims, although 1 drachm is a very common dose, and in some cases 4 drachms or 1 oz. may be given with impunity.

Another instance :—

Pil. coloc. co.   .   .   .   .   .   . gr. ij.
Pil. cambogiæ co. .   .   .   .   .   . gr. j.
Strychninæ .   .   .   .   .   . gr. $\frac{1}{24}$
Ext. bellad. .   .   .   .   .   . gr. ij.

Ft. pil. in arg.   Mitte xxiv.   Sig.   One at bedtime.

Two grains of ext. bellad. for a dose is unusual, but, since it was for an adult and only exhibited once a day, it might have been dispensed. But the dispenser happened to know that the prescriber gave only *small* doses of belladonna ; he was therefore consulted, and the dose altered to $\frac{1}{4}$ of a grain.

We know of another case in which an M.D. ordered ext. belladonnæ q.s. to make a mass, and *he meant it.* The quantity required varied in his prescriptions, and his pharmacist made it a rule never to give more than 1 grain.

Where unusual doses are prescribed, the quantity should be indicated in words as well as figures. No emphasising of a badly written or smudged figure will render it less ambiguous ; but if it be indicated in both ways it is scarcely possible that there could be any doubt of the interpretation. Thus—

> Tr. opii   .   .   .   . m L. (50 minims) h.s.s.

would save the dispenser from any hesitation as to whether the quantity was L. or 4.

Extra Doses.—In the German Pharmacopœia a table of maximum doses of certain powerful medicines is given, and if the prescriber desire to exceed the quantities there set down he is required to mark the quantity. If this be not done the dispenser is held responsible for the consequences if he dispense the dangerous dose. Two curious cases are mentioned by Dr. Hager. In one, an extra dose of cyanide of potassium had been ordered, and the prescriber had several times *underlined* the quantity. The patient died, and the dispenser was condemned to a year's imprisonment because he had dispensed the medicine without the proper mark (!) being attached. In the other case, the physician meant to order 4 grammes of chloral hydrate, and he should have written grm. 4·0. He omitted the decimal point, however, and the dispenser gave 40 grammes. At that time chloral hydrate was not included in the German Pharmacopœia, and therefore was not in the table of dangerous substances. But the dispenser was sentenced to a long term of imprisonment.

It is indeed a constantly recurring difficulty to dispensers of limited experience to know whether certain quantities prescribed are not either unusual or dangerous doses. The Pharmacopœia ceases to be a guide, for individual prescribers entertain varying ideas respecting the potency of drugs. A prescriber, especially if eminent in his particular line, will not consent to initial in such cases, or to add any indication of unusual dose. He resents the fact that his method of prescribing should not be familiar to the dispenser. Quinine sulphate is ordered occasionally in heroic doses ; and, as regards the salts of morphine—especially the acetate—opium and its preparations, it would be difficult to say where the maximum limit ends. A provincial dispenser may always feel safe when the autograph prescription bears the business stamp of some London house. The recipe has probably been dispensed many times ; and the pharmacist is advised not to indicate by his manner, still less by any direct question to the patient, that there appears to him to be anything remarkable in the formula which he is called upon to dispense.

But do not follow the example of the London house if you think that there is a chance of poisoning the patient. For instance, a prescription was given in to a provincial house which ordered a large dose (about an ounce) of aq. laurocerasi. It bore the stamp of a leading London house, and appeared therefore to have been taken by the patient with safety. Not being satisfied, inquiry was made, and it was found that the firm referred to had, in dispensing the recipe, omitted a considerable quantity of the aq. laurocer. (the writer was a provincial doctor and could not, of course, be consulted). This emphasises the aphorism : If a prescription be altered it should be so marked.

Many examples of large doses could be cited. Two grains of extract. cannabis indicæ have been given every two hours in a case of tetanus, but the case was watched by several medical men. Dr. Heron Watson (of Edinburgh) regularly prescribes teaspoonful doses of subnitrate of bismuth. In some cases ordinary doses of narcotics cause great excitement. For example, 30 grains of chloral have made a man most obstreperous, but drachm doses induced sleep. A well-known authority states that he has seen 5 oz. of the juice of conium ordered and taken daily, $\frac{1}{2}$ grain of pure hyoscyamine for a dose ; 1 drachm of tincture of Indian hemp three times a day ; also $\frac{1}{2}$ lb. of mercury for a dose. The patients who took these doses were, of course, under special observation.

The following prescription was given to dispense as a draught :—

Potass. iodid. .	.	.	.	.	.	.	ʒiss.
Tr. aurantii .	.	.	.	.	.	.	ʒij.
Tr. cinchonæ .	.	.	.	.	.	.	℥ss.

M.

No directions were given. On the pharmacist expostulating with the customer as to the largeness of the dose of iodide, it was most strenuously affirmed that it was for one dose only. It had been dispensed before for a friend, who lent it to the customer. This lending of prescriptions often leads to bad results and should not be encouraged.

General Directions are as a rule unsatisfactory and often lead to mistakes. We have been asked, If a doctor sends a prescription for a mixture (not dangerous) marked 'Special : *To be taken as directed*,' is he justified in condemning the dispenser as an unpardonable offender for sending the mixture to the patient without further instructions respecting dose ?

'To be taken as directed' implies that the prescriber has given directions, but it is not uncommon to find that the prescriber has omitted to give directions, and for that reason it is always safe for the dispenser to ask the customer how the medicine is to be used, and so ascertain whether the directions are sufficient or not. If the mixture is dangerous it is safe to see the doctor. The prescriber was not justified in censuring the chemist as above stated.

Errors in the Prescription.—If possible, reference should be made to the writer. Caution must be used in concluding that a *fancied* error or omission is *real*. 'Common sense' is frequently appealed to, but this indefinable judge cannot be called into operation unless the 'sense of the community' on the point in question has been obtained. Too many people confound their own individual opinion with the dictates of 'common sense.' For instance, some dispensers invariably add acid to a mixture containing quinine, although solution of the alkaloid is not prescribed. Now, many physicians prefer administering quinine *in suspension*, and it is decidedly less disagreeable taken in this manner, especially when large doses are exhibited. Moreover, when quinine is given to a woman nursing it is usual on the part of the prescriber to avoid an acid, as it checks the secretion of milk.

Wishes of Patients—On this point Dr. Whitla says, 'Where a prescription is repeatedly compounded the patient often asks for the dose to be increased, or some other change to be made. The dispenser should not accede to such a request, no matter how simple it may appear, without a consultation with the prescriber ; nor is it advisable for him to inform the patient (even when pressed) of the ingredients in any prescription. He can refer them to the physician, or do as the writer has done long ago, when it was impossible to avoid such a revelation—read it in full Latin to the patient.' This ruling is somewhat stringent. One frequently meets with customers— they are generally regular customers—who may safely get a hint as to what a medicine is composed of.

Repeating Prescriptions.—There is no rule against repeating a prescription as often as may be desired by the patient, but a conscientious regard should be had in such cases to his ultimate good. The majority of prescriptions, fortunately, may be repeated without warning or comment ; but there are some, such as those containing arsenic, digitalis, strychnine, &c., which, from their cumulative tendency, may produce serious consequences if repeated too frequently ; and in such cases it is, we believe, not more to the interest of the patient than the dispenser that the suggestion be made to again consult the physician as to their continuance. There are other prescriptions, such as those containing chloral, morphine, and other narcotics, the repetition of which is apt to engender the worst of vices on the part of the patient. A little reflection will show the responsibility incurred where repetition may lead to the formation of a bad habit.

SPECIAL DRUGS AND DISPENSING CONVENIENCES.

WATERS.

Aqua.—There is no longer any ambiguity as to what is meant when 'aqua' is ordered in a prescription, for the British Pharmacopœia (1885) explicitly states : ' In dispensing prescriptions, *aqua* should be understood to mean distilled water.' Distilled water, according to the Pharmacopœia, is made by taking ten gallons of water and distilling it from a copper still with block-tin worm, rejecting the first half-gallon and collecting the next eight gallons. It is distinguished from ordinary water by containing no solid constituent, and should be free from ammonia when tested by Nessler's solution.

As supplies of distilled water are generally obtained from wholesale houses it should never be stocked without examining it. Frequently it is simply the condensed vapour from steam-heating pipes or steam boilers ; consequently it is liable to contain impurities. Ammonia and nitrites are the most common, the latter giving very strange results in mixtures containing iodides. Moreover, such distilled water has a tendency to become viscous, owing to the formation of thread-like organisms. The surest plan is to distil water as it is required, adding to each gallon of water in the still ten grains of permanganate of potash and a drachm of sulphuric acid. This ensures the destruction of organic matter, the products of which remain in the still.

Aqua fontana should not be used unless when ordered. The varying quantity of calcareous matter which different natural waters contain is alone a sufficient reason for excluding them from the dispensing counter, because some mixtures compounded with such water differ in appearance according to the amount of calcareous matter contained in the water. The following are examples of what may be expected when distilled water and spring water are used indifferently.

Tinct. lavand. co. gives a bright mixture with distilled, but a muddy one with tap water. Tinct. cardamom. co. produces with distilled water a reddish-brown colour, but with tap water a brilliant crimson, as though ammonia had been added.

Liq. arsenicalis gives a precipitate of calcium carbonate with tap water, which will probably be regarded by the nervous patient as the arsenic imperfectly dissolved, if it has been previously obtained without such a deposit owing to the use of distilled water.

If a prescription containing liq. hydrarg. perchlor. and water be dispensed with distilled water a clear mixture is obtained ; if common water is used a precipitate consisting of an insoluble mercury salt is thrown down.

Such prescriptions as the following are constantly seen at the dispensing-counter :—

I.

Argent. nit.	.	.	.	gr. v.
Aquæ	.	.	.	ℨj.
Mix.				

II.

Syr. ferri iod.	.	.	.	ℨj.
Aquæ	.	.	.	ad ℥iv.
Mix.				

III.

Plumbi acet.	.	.	.	gr. xij.
Sp. vin. rect.	.	.	.	ℨj.
Aquæ	.	.	.	ad ℥iv.
Mix.				

IV.

Ammon. carb.	.	.	ℨss
Spir. chlorof.	.	.	ℨj.
Inf. gent. co.	.	.	.	℥vj.
Mix.				

In many cases it is advisable even to boil the distilled water, for if it happen to contain carbonic acid or atmospheric air, decomposition will be accelerated. I. and II. are good examples. It may also be remarked that in dispensing III. the rectified spirit should be mixed with the water before the acetate of lead is dissolved in it. The spirit furthers the expulsion of the air and carbonic acid gas, which are mostly present if the distilled water is not fresh.

If the infusion of gentian in No. 4 be made with plain water, the result will be that the lime mostly present in ordinary water, and which is only deposited on prolonged boiling, coming in contact with the ammonia will render the mixture slightly turbid, and give a deposit of calcium carbonate on the sides of the bottle.

Extemporaneous Aromatic Waters.—Distilled aromatic waters have a finer flavour than those prepared by the mixture method, and in some cases, notably rose water, the odour of the extemporaneous preparation is of quite a different character from the distilled. Various substances of an alkaline-earthy nature are added to the oils in the mixture method in order to render them soluble, and, as has been shown by Shuttleworth, these substances generally keep back a portion of the oil, so that the water takes up no more, or little more, than it would do if the earthy powder were not added. It should also be remembered that the powder dissolves to some extent, and therefore affects mixtures containing alkaloids and other substances precipitable by alkalies. This may be obviated by the adoption of either of the following processes.

In the official process of the United States Pharmacopœia the essential oil is directed to be added to a proper quantity of cotton wool, teasing and mixing the wool thoroughly, and then packing tightly in a percolator and pouring on the necessary amount of water. The amount of oil used in most cases is 1 part to 500 of water (say a drop to the ounce). In the ‘Art of Pharmacy’ we have published a method which is very simple, and gives excellent products. In this an excess of oil is used, the reason being that the excess gives much finer waters than are obtained by using a less amount. Prepare a solution of 6 fluid drachms of essential oil in 4 fluid ounces of rectified spirit (60 o.p.) and of this add 1 ounce to 4 pnits of water. Shake well, and allow to stand until clear, then syphon off the clear water.

D

The earthy powders which are most used for rendering essential oils soluble are light carbonate of magnesia, powdered pumice stone, kaolin, silica, phosphate of calcium and talc (French chalk). The method to be followed for a pint of any water is to dissolve from 20 to 40 minims of the oil in four times as much spirit, add an ounce of water, and triturate with half an ounce of any of the powders (2 drachms of magnes. carb. levis is enough). The most objectionable powder is magnesia, and the least objectionable is talc. The following excellent method of using the latter has been proposed.

Wash finely pulverised white talc with hot water slightly acidulated with hydrochloric acid, and finally with hot water only to remove acid, then dry and stock for use. The powder may be used by adding half an ounce of it to the cloudy mixture (such as is formed by shaking up ℥ss. of ol. anethi and ℥ij. of S.V.R. in a quart of water), and filtering through paper, or a *talc filter* may be prepared in the following manner: Make a double filter out of white filtering-paper and insert it in a quart glass funnel; mix about half an ounce of talc with one pint of hot water in a bottle, shake well and pour upon the filter, taking care to so distribute the mixture that the entire filter from bottom to top is evenly covered with the fine powder; the water will rapidly pass off perfectly clear, after which the filter is ready for filtering any cloudy mixture. The same filter may be used frequently for the same substances. After using it, cover the funnel with a glass plate to exclude dust and preserve it for the next operation.

Camphor water may be made quickly by dissolving ℥iiss. of spt. camph. B.P. in 40 oz. of water.

CONCENTRATED INFUSIONS.

In most of the large establishments the duty of preparing infusions for use during the day falls to the assistant who has been on night duty. Without discussing the question whether the dispenser is justified in using concentrated infusions or not, it may be said that, strictly speaking, the pharmacist should use only freshly prepared infusions. An experienced pharmacist says on this point, 'Never use concentrated infusions when time allows of fresh ones being made. The aroma of the recent infusion is often wanting, whilst the difference in appearance is in most cases very marked.'

The subject has been very fully discussed in the 'Art of Pharmacy,' and a process there given for making concentrated preparations which equal fresh ones in aroma, etc. There are one or two infusions which should always be prepared fresh, notably infusion of digitalis. Dr. Hager has given this infusion as one which may be used concentrated, but it is the very one which many therapeutists state should not be kept in the concentrated state. Fresh infusion of digitalis is, in fact, the most active and reliable preparation of the drug.

When 8 oz. of any infusion are required, 10 oz. at least should be made, as the marc absorbs a good deal of the menstruum, and the Pharmacopœia does not direct it to be pressed out.

SOLUTIONS.

It is usual for dispensers to keep solutions of salts often required in prescriptions. These are not only convenient, but frequently impart to a mixture a bright appearance which otherwise would be wanting. No one would recognise a mixture made with infus. rosæ acid. and Epsom salts in solution as the same preparation if made by the addition of the salts. The same is true, in greater or less degree, of very many other previously made solutions ; to a large extent this accounts for the physical differences observed in mixtures dispensed at different establishments.

The following are the solutions which are in most common use in large establishments. It should be noted that solids for any quantity in ounces should be taken by troy weight— that is, 480 grains ; for example, sol. ammon. brom. 1 in 4 means 480 grs. ammon. brom. in 4 fl. oz. of the solution.

Sol. Acid Tannic	. . . . . .	1 in 2 (S.V.R.)
,, Aluminis .	. . . . .	1 in 16
,, Ammonii bromidi	. . . .	1 in 4
,, Ferri tartarat. .	. . . . .	1 in 4

Sol. Ferri et quininæ citrat.	.	.	.	.	1 in 2
,, Magnesii sulphatis		.	.	.	1 in 2
,, Potassii acetatis	.	.	.	.	1 in 2
,, ,, bicarbonatis .	.	.	.	.	1 in 4
,, ,, nitratis	.	.	.	.	1 in 8
,, ,, chloratis	.	.	.	.	1 in-24
,, ,, bromidi	.	.	.	.	1 in 4
,, ,, iodidi .	.	.	.	.	1 in 2
,, Plumbi acetatis	.	.	.	.	1 in 16
,, Sodii bicarbonatis	.	.	.	.	1 in 16
,, Zinci chloridi	.	.	.	.	1 in 4
,, ,, sulphatis .	.	.	.	.	1 in 8

The solutions of bicarbonates are liable to become somewhat changed with formation of carbonate, with the result that mixtures containing vegetable colouring-matter are much darkened ; such solutions also precipitate magnesia from the sulphate. It is a good plan to keep all these dispensing solutions in a dark cupboard ; many of them are affected by light.

The following remarks on dispensing solutions and the way to prepare them should have the attention of the dispenser.

Dr. Hager states that *iodide of potassium* solution (1 in 2) does not keep well, and recommends that only so much should be made as will keep for eight or ten days in a dark place, and that it should only be dispensed if quite clear and colourless. *Potassio-tartrate of antimony* (1 in 50) is also sometimes kept in solution, and this too spoils in a short time, but the addition of ʒi. of S.V.R. to each pint is helpful.

We may, however, remark that in many instances concentrated solutions keep much better than weaker solutions. Quinine and iron citrate is a notable example, a solution of 1 part in 2 keeping for weeks, while a weaker solution quickly becomes bad.

In weak solution chloral hydrate soon decomposes and becomes acid, acquiring an odour not unlike a mixture of tolu and benzene. We prefer not to keep this chemical in solution, but in powder form, so that it dissolves readily.

Scale Preparations can with care be readily and easily dissolved in the bottle in which they are to be dispensed. A little of the water or aqueous vehicle should be put into the bottle first, being careful not to wet its neck ; or, should this be done, it should be dried with a cloth, else the scale preparation will adhere to this moisture and block the admission of the salt into the bottle. A solution is readily formed if the salt falls upon the water and is quickly agitated—not allowed to 'cake' at the bottom.

There are exceptions to every rule, however, and the slow solubility and extreme frothiness on agitation of sulphate of beberine marks it out as a very decided exception to the other scale preparations. The better plan with this salt is to rub it down into fine powder in the mortar, then add water with constant stirring so as to prevent it forming into an adhesive mass on either mortar or pestle. If this be done properly it will dissolve quickly and without the least trouble ; if any other plan be tried it will certainly cake and cause no end of trouble. A few drops of ac. sulph. dil. may be added.

Ferrum tartaratum dissolves with difficulty in cold, but very readily in hot, water. The most satisfactory method of manipulation is to put it in a dry mortar and pour hot water over it, when it goes down with the least possible trouble. With distilled water it gives a perfectly clear solution, but with tap water the solution never becomes clear.

CONCENTRATED MIXTURES, &c.

Mist. Ammoniaci Conc., 1 in 7.—This may be made by emulsifying 1 part of ammoniacum with 4 parts of water. For use add 1 part to 7 parts of water.

Mist. Cretæ Co.—The powders for chalk mixture may be kept ready mixed, so that 1 oz. of the mixture with 7½ oz. of cinnamon water will make mist. cretæ co., B.P.

Mist. Ferri Co.—The emulsion should be kept ready made, and the iron added only at the time of using.

Syr. Ferri Iodidi.—This is now largely prepared from the liquor, which is kept permanently bright and free from oxidation by means of a trace of hypophosphorus acid. Many syrups which are rarely required and which are apt to decompose on keeping may be prepared from the liquors, provided the dispenser assures himself that the finished product is similar to the official one in strength, etc.

There are many other preparations which may be conveniently kept in the concentrated or 'liquor' form. Some manfacturers have made this class of preparations a speciality It would be out of place to speak of their products here, but it may be said that if the dispenser is seldom called upon for certain preparations, such as syrups, which on keeping undergo apparent alteration, these may be kept in stock in the permanent 'liquor' form, to be diluted as required. The dispenser should, of course, satisfy himself that the product answers to the official requirements.

SPECIAL DRUGS AND CHEMICALS.

Acacia in mixtures is best used in the form of mucilage in the proper proportion. Gum Senegal, according to Hager, has an unpleasant taste and smell, and acts chemically with the metallic salts ; so it should not be used instead of the true gum. Care should be taken that the mucilage is fresh. It quickly sours, and we have seen curious and often puzzling complications from this cause.

Heat applied in making mucilage of acacia is an ingenious method o producing a bad preparation for the sake of saving time. Powdered gum should only be used in making emulsions (which see). The practice has been adopted in first-class dispensing establishments of employing only small picked gum, allowing it to macerate in the water till dissolved, but aiding the solution by occasional stirring with a bone spatula. Strain through muslin. This mucilage will keep any reasonable length of time, and is remarkably clear and bright.

Camphor, when not wanted as an emulsion, may be mixed in water or in any aqueous menstruum in the following manner : Make a definite solution (A) of camphor, the more concentrated the better, in sp. vini rect. Make a second spirituous solution (B) of equal parts of S.V.R. and distilled water. Allow the mixture to stand so as to become perfectly cool. Add the camphorated alcohol (A) in any fixed proportion, say 1 : 4 or 1 : 8, to the quasi-proof spirit (B). The resulting essence will be found miscible with water ; and the dose of camphor may be accurately administered.

Glycerine is a useful and powerful solvent, acting at the same time as an antiseptic. It is largely used as a sweetening agent in mixtures, especially those containing perchloride of iron. It is the best and most appropriate solvent and preservative of the peptic and pancreatic ferments, and is added to tincture of kino in order to prevent gelatinisation. Pill-masses containing a little glycerine do not harden, but care must be taken to avoid excess, as too much makes the pills hygroscopic. For dispensing it is best kept diluted with an equal volume of water, as then it is easily poured, and there is less loss from part of it remaining in the measure.

Iodine only slightly dissolves in water, but iodide of potassium would make three-quarters of its own weight soluble. Ammonia salts also increase its solubility owing to the formation of ammonium iodide. Oils of peppermint and fennel, and some other volatile oils, combine chemically with iodine. When iodine occurs in a prescription without any solvent see the prescriber, and suggest the addition of sufficient iodide of potassium to dissolve the iodine.

Manna is occasionally wanted in a state of solution in an English prescription. In Continental dispensing its use is more frequent, especially amongst German prescribers. Direct heat should never be applied to effect its solution. Allow the manna to macerate in just as much cold water as will change it into a soft pasty mass; then add the rest of the water required and dissolve by a gentle heat. Strain through fine muslin. Time and trouble will be saved by this process, and the manna will not crystallise out of the solution, as would otherwise be the case. When manna is present in excess, and can only be partially suspended, as occurs in several foreign formulæ, previous cold maceration is still the best mode of proceeding.

Morphine Salts should be dissolved without heat, for at a temperature above 40° C. (104° F.), their solutions are apt to turn yellowish or even brown. With care beautiful solutions may be made. The meconate of morphine is affected least, but this solution should only be filtered through paper which has previously been washed free from iron by means of hydrochloric acid and water, otherwise the solution will be coloured red.

Quinine Sulphate for dispensing purposes should be reduced to powder ; the bulk is much diminished, and trouble is obviated whenever the sulphate has to be exhibited in a pilular form. It is more easily weighed. A solution of 5 parts in 90 parts of distilled water and 5 parts of diluted sulphuric acid is sometimes kept in solution. A fungoid growth, the mycelium of a fungus, probably penicilium, is formed, but it is doubtful if this is at the expense of the quinine. Certainly any diminution of strength is inappreciable, and this applies to solutions of most alkaloids. The addition of 5 per cent. of rectified spirit prevents the growth of the fungus in the case of quinine solution ; so also does a trace of chloroform.

If a prescription contain nothing in which the quinine may be dissolved, it should be merely rubbed down and sent out with a ' shake the bottle ' label. It is taking an unwarrantable and unnecessary liberty to add any acid whatever, and the same may be said regarding the addition of mucilage. If you know that the prescriber wishes acid to be added, do so and note the fact on the prescription.

Never dissolve quinine sulphate with hydrochloric acid if that acid is not ordered ; such a solution is not fluorescent, and if the prescription happens to have been dispensed before with sulphuric acid, the patient may notice the difference, and draw an inference. Quinine is largely prescribed on the Continent in combination with extract of liquorice. In this case first dissolve the extract in ten times its weight of water, then add the solution of quinine, as both the alkaloid and the acid tend to throw out a dirty-looking precipitate of glycyrrhizin.

When quinine and liquorice are prescribed together without acid, and it is found necessary to make any addition to produce a presentable mixture, acacia or tragacanth should be used.

Spt. Ætheris Nitrosi very quickly decomposes and becomes acid, and requires to be made alkaline with bicarbonate of potash before being compounded with bromide or iodide of potassium, otherwise free bromine or iodine will be liberated, and the mixture darkened. Some dispensers keep a crystal or two of bicarbonate of potash in the spirit, and thus have it always neutral, but that of course does not prevent decomposition of the nitrous ether: nitrite of the alkali is really formed.

Silver Nitrate in solution should be sent out in amber-tinted or uranium glass bottles, which more effectually prevent the actinic action of light on the solution, and being more transparent than blue-glass bottles they enable the patient to see what he has in the bottle more clearly.

Sugar.—When prescribed in mixtures use simple syrup, as clear solutions of sugar can only be made on the application of heat. For every ounce avoirdupois of sugar use 9 fluid drachms of syrup; or for every drachm of sugar use 68 minims.

Tannic Acid will easily dissolve in pure water, yielding a solution with a light yellow shade. The water must be quite free from ammonia, or the solution gradually darkens to a brownish tint. With traces of iron it turns inky, and alkaline substances also turn it thick and brown to black. With mucilages of carragheen, salep, althæa, etc., it forms flaky conglomerates, and should only be mixed with them after dilution with twenty times its weight of water.

PILLS AND THEIR EXCIPIENTS.

GENERAL OBSERVATIONS.

THE preparation of good pills often requires much practical judgment and experience, and is, indeed, one of the most important parts of pharmacy, for it is here that the prescriber leaves much to the superior knowledge of the pharmacist.

The characteristics of well-prepared pills are that they are not too soft, do not stick together nor flatten, that they are smooth and round, all of the same size, and all contain similar proportions of the ingredients. As far as possible it is advisable to send out pills of the same weight as prescribed, and since inspissation is more or less inconvenient at the dispensing-counter, this object is attained by keeping the more common extracts both in a soft condition and in a state sufficiently hard to roll into pills with but little addition of powder. Ext. coloc. co. and ext. rhei are more conveniently kept in the state of powder, as also are several pill-masses—*e.g.* pil. asafœt. co., pil. cambog. co., pil. aloes et ferri, pil. aloes et myrrhæ, pil. hyd. subchlor. co., etc. State clearly on the label how much of the pill mass the powder is equivalent to; for example—'Pulv. pro pil. hydrarg. subchlor. co., 4 grains equal 5 grains of pill mass.'

Before rolling out the mass into pills it is a good plan to weigh it in order to see that it corresponds with the total weight of the ingredients. This is a good precaution, and especially checks careless weighing. Unless the prescriber order to the contrary, it is advisable to make up to 1 grain all pills less than that in weight. This is done by adding some inert powder, such as liquorice or sugar of milk with an appropriate excipient, and if a note is kept in the prescription-book of the size of the pills, which should invariably be done, it ensures the same sized pill always being sent. Great care should be taken that pills dispensed at one time should not differ in size from the same dispensed on another occasion. Note remark under German prescriptions, that in Germany pills are seldom prescribed more than about 2 grains each in weight, and this also is the tendency of English pharmacy.

Where no excipient is ordered the simplest should be selected, and that which gives least increase to the size of the pill. Generally speaking, a dispenser has one excipient that he prefers and uses in the majority of cases. It may not be the best in every case, but, because he is in the habit of using it, and knows well its massing powers, he can produce better results with it than with any other. Citrate of iron and quinine, for example, may be made into a good working mass and keeping pill with almost any excipient not having glycerine for its basis; but if a dispenser tries to make a mass with any excipient other than that which he is in the habit of using, the chances are that the attempt will end, at least in the first instance, in failure. It is necessary to point this out, as in none of the cases afterwards mentioned would we consider the excipients recommended the best unless this element of familiarity in their use were also taken into consideration.

Rolling.—In small establishments where a 4 or 5 grain pill machine is the only apparatus of that kind available, it is a matter of difficulty to roll out a mass for 1 or 2 grain pills upon the large machine. To meet this disadvantage a correspondent of *The Chemist and Druggist* states that he uses a pill-roller resembling the figure on next page. The advantages of this little instrument are apparent. It should be about 3 inches broad, but it can be made any length less than the breadth of the machine. The roller should be made of hard wood—such as walnut—and the handle is securely fixed into the bottom piece with glue.

Another good idea for a roller is a piece of beech wood about ⅜ inch thick, 6 inches long, and 4 inches broad. A leather strap is nailed to each side, and goes across the top. Under this four fingers of the hand are placed, and the thumb fits on one side to steady it. For working up masses or rolling weighed portions into pipe it is capital, because the pressure can be applied as desired.

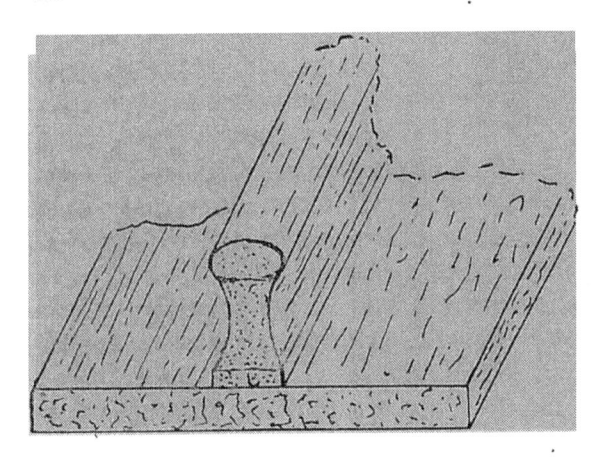

Still another idea has been put forward. It is to insert into the bed of the machine a piece of mahogany board (about ⅛ inch thick) made the required size, so that it may slip into the machine and be a tight fit. By this arrangement the ordinary roller can be used, and 1 grain pills are rolled out quite easily.

Rounding.—Pills are generally rounded with a pill-rounder. Rounding pills with the fingers is only permissible when the mass is of such a character that it crumbles under the rounder. The ordinary rounder has a deep and a shallow side, so that large and small sizes may be rounded in it ; but if either side is too deep, the insertion of a piece of cardboard is useful. The engraving on page 46 shows the parts of a French pill-roller (Vial's *Disque à pilules*) which can be put together to suit any ordinary size. The cut pills are laid on the tray, sprinkled with a little powder, and, being covered by the roller, they are rapidly, and with slight pressure, revolved.

Powder is used to prevent pills sticking to each other, and, 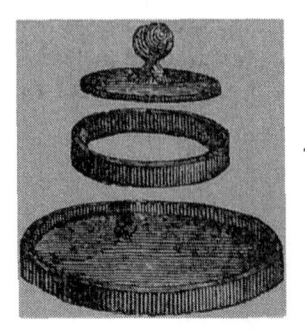 to some extent, to conceal their taste. When no particular powder is ordered, lycopodium is used in Germany ; but this is inadmissible in Great Britain. A mixture of starches, cinnamon, liquorice, magnes. carb. levis, and powdered French chalk are all used —the latter, perhaps, more than any other. The objection to it is that it makes the slab very slippery; but this can be overcome by the addition of a little powdered starch. A pill-sieve is sometimes employed to remove excess of powder.

Pills with hygroscopic, strong-smelling, or volatile ingredients should always be dispensed in bottles.

To make pills that will keep their shape for a reasonable time they ought to contain some fibrous vegetable powder in their composition. Where such is not ordered the dispenser has often to use it, but, of course, what he uses must be both medicinally and chemically inert. Paper-pulp—blotting-paper or filtering-paper scraped into fluff—has also been recommended.

Small quantities of ingredients, such as a fraction of a grain of a powerful medicament (strychnine, perchloride of mercury, calcium sulphide, etc.), should be intimately mixed with sugar of milk and massed with soft manna. Sugar of milk, in *crystals*, or coarse powder, is most useful for dividing any active ingredient when making pills. A mortar and pestle with perfectly smooth grinding-surfaces should be selected, and the strychnine (for example) lightly powdered ; an equal quantity of coarse sugar of milk should be added, and lightly triturated until none adheres to the mortar ; then powder carefully, add a little more coarse sugar of milk, triturate lightly until mixed and detached from the mortar, then powder, and mix thoroughly with any other powders that may be ordered in the pill.

Hot-plate.—A small water-bath or a small hot-water plate should be at hand for evaporating pills to suitable consistence, adding a little tragacanth, if necessary. Many operations in pill-making, especially when large masses are on hand, are greatly facilitated by the use of a *smooth slab of iron*, say 9 inches square of $\frac{1}{4}$ inch boiler plate ; it is quickly warmed over a gas furnace, and as soon as the plate is hot enough (as may be judged by the finger) the gas is put out, and the mass placed upon it.

Pills containing much aloes, colocynth (pill or extract), asafœtida, or galbanum, being so liable to fall, should be made with its assistance. Black pitch, solid chian turpentine, and some other substances hard and brittle in the cold, may be rolled on the hot iron slab and made into pills without addition of a liquid excipient, but some require fibrous material, such as liquorice powder or lycopodium, in order to prevent their falling.

Substances which are decomposed by iron, such as corrosive sublimate, calomel, nitrate of silver, copper and bismuth salts, must not be mixed in an iron mortar. Salts easily soluble in water naturally require very careful addition of moisture, and excipients containing glycerine should be avoided, or used very sparingly.

Soft Masses.—Crystallised salts, fluid acids, soft extracts, with an organic powder, often make a mass of muddy consistence, which rights itself by waiting ten to fifteen minutes. Time should always be given for an organic powder to suck up moisture. For soft masses a desiccator, such as that in use for drying precipitates, etc., in the laboratory, is a most useful adjunct to the dispensing-counter. A very soft mass, cut into pills, and these dried by placing in a desiccator over strong sulphuric acid for twelve hours, has frequently turned out well. This treatment is especially applicable when pills contain deliquescent salts.

Liquid excipients.—The drawing on next page shows a dropping-bottle, called 'Salleron's drop-counter,' which is useful for adding water to pill-masses. A Maw's eye-drop bottle and a Chalk's drop-bottle are very useful for dropping small quantities of water or spirit into a pill-mass.

In well-appointed establishments several bottles containing syrup, mucilage, glycerine and water, and other fluids, are kept

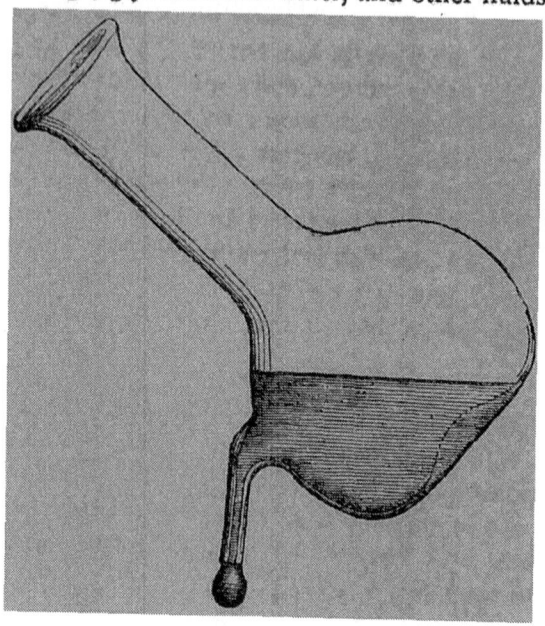

on the dispensing-counter. The figure (p. 49) shows a suitable bottle.

Where fluids require to be added to form a pill-mass, it will always be found risky to add them direct to the mass; and as a dropper may not be available, a good plan is to drop the fluid first on to the point of the spatula, and from it to the mortar in quantity necessary to form a mass.

Pill-masses containing dry vegetable powders require some few minutes to absorb the added water, and therefore should be made softish, and allowed to stand for ten to fifteen minutes before rolling, or they are liable to crumble. If the exact quantity of water or syrup required for massing a powder be known, the pills may be made of smaller size, and in less time, by adding the required quantity at once, and rapidly mixing and cutting before the absorption has caused too much firmness.

The addition of the excipient little by little generally adds much to the labour, and not infrequently much also to the size of the pills. This applies to excipients such as extracts as well as to liquids. Never use the same spatula to scrape the mass from the pestle and to dip into the extract-pot.

If the quantity of extract ordered would make the mass too soft, the dispenser must, if the extract be an active one, either use it in a drier state or add some inert powder to it. If the extract, however, be of no particular activity, Dr. Hager says that some powder of the same plant may be substituted for a portion of it—as, for instance, if 20 grains of extract of gentian were ordered, one might use 10 grains of extract with 10 grains of powdered gentian.

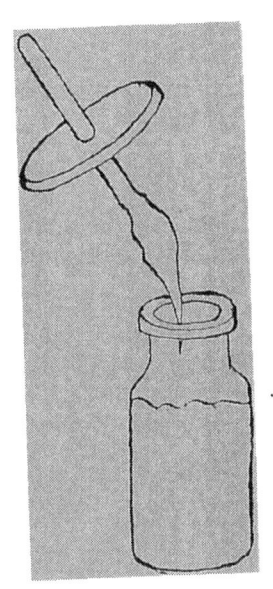

AN EMPTY 1 OZ. CITRATE OF IRON AND QUININE BOTTLE.

The cover made of sheet india-rubber, a little larger than the mouth of the bottle, and the dipping-rod of glass.

The objection to this plan is the variation which is apt to arise in the size of the pills, 10 grains of an extract and 10 grains of the crude powder frequently producing an objectionable increase in the bulk of the pill. The better plan, we think, in such cases, is to diminish rather than increase the bulk of the pill, and therefore when an extract is too soft, we recommend that it be evaporated to a proper consistence ; and for this reason every pharmacist should have some simple and ready appliance for accomplishing this without risk to the extract. When extracts are evaporated, regard must always be had to the hygroscopic qualities of some of them, otherwise the pills may become semi-fluid in the patient's keeping.

E

INGREDIENTS OF PILLS AND HOW TO MASS THEM.

Acetate of Potash, which seems one of the most unreasonable things to put into a pill, makes, according to Whitla, a good mass with Canada balsam, and remains stable. A more desirable mass is obtained with boro-tartrate of potash—*e.g.* acetate of potash 18 parts, boro-tartrate of potash 3 parts, and water 1 part, can be made into pills without much difficulty and keep well in corked bottles.

Acids.—The mineral acids are rarely, if ever, prescribed in pill form in this country, but it sometimes happens that a German prescription of this nature turns up. With the addition of marshmallow powder and glycerinated water good plastic masses are obtained, as in the following :—

							Grammes
Pepsini	.	.	.	.	.	.	2·5
Rad. rhei	.	.	.	.	.	.	5·0
Extr. gentianæ	.	.	.	.	.	.	1·5
Acid. muriatici	.	.	.	.	.	gtt.	20

(Rad. alth., aq. glycerini, each 0·5.)

M.   Ft. pilulæ 100.

Send out such pills in a bottle.

Acidum Benzoicum—Five grains make a fair mass with a drop of glycerine, but Canada balsam generally gives better results, especially if the balsam is new and thin.

Acidum Gallicum makes a good mass with a sixth to an eighth of its weight of glycerine.

Aloes.—Pills containing aloes in any fair proportion, and particularly when in combination with colocynth, scammony, and soap, are best made with decoct. aloes comp., which an eminent pharmacist has called their 'natural excipient.' It has great solvent power, and must be used in very sparing quantity. The many compounds of aloes, mastic, and soap, in varying proportions, are best made with this excipient, but the dispenser must guard against chemical action. Dec. aloes co. owes its value as an excipient chiefly to the presence of carbonate of potassium, which is an active solvent of organic substances, but not in every case a desirable addition to a pillmass. Aloes alone is the better for the addition of some fibrous material, and if massed with mucilage of acacia and rolled out quickly, the pills keep their shape very well. Large masses should be made with the assistance of a hot plate.

Antipyrin.—Use 1 grain of tragacanth for each 5 grains, and mass with as little water as possible.

Balsams, Oils, etc.—Pill-masses are sometimes required with fluid or soft resins, fluid balsams, oils, or fats, as ingredients. When the quantity of these is too large to admit of the formation of a mass by the addition of any reasonable quantity of powder, recourse must be had to wax. Balsam of Peru, copaiba, extract of male fern, oleo-resin of cubebs, creosote, carbolic acid, ethereal oils, and other substances, melted by a gentle heat with one-third to an equal weight of wax, yield, according to Dr. Hager, very good pill-masses, but the mixture must be quite cold before combination with any other ingredients. The addition of ether or spirit destroys the plasticity of this compound. The wax, with the medicament, must be melted very slowly in a porcelain dish, as the application of a strong heat would be likely to injure the medicinal properties of the ingredients. In using wax the dispenser must be careful that he does not bring the resulting mass to such a degree of hardness that the pills will not disintegrate in the alimentary canal. This is the great objection to the use of wax. An ordinary pill, though much harder than a wax pill, may dissolve in the stomach, because its ingredients are soluble in water. Wax pills are generally insoluble in water.

Balsam Peru is seldom ordered alone in pills. The following formula may be adopted when so ordered : Bals. Peru, gr. xxx., slaked lime (in fine powder), gr. xv., castor oil and rectified spirit, of each two drops. This forms a mass which remains soft, and is of good pilular consistence. It requires to stand for an hour before being rolled out.

The following prescription shows a difficulty :—

Ferri redact.	gr. iij.
Bals. Peru	♏ ss.
Pulv. amyli q.s. ut fiat pil.	
Mitte 36.	

Starch-powder is not the best absorbent in this case, because it is too gritty for pill-masses and rather retards than aids the binding of the mass. Liquorice-powder is much better. After rubbing the reduced iron to ensure fineness of division, the balsam and half its weight of treacle are added, and well beaten together. The resulting mass is soft and oily in appearance, but not crumbly, and the addition of liquorice-powder, q.s., gives the required stiffness. The small percentage of alkali in the treacle seems to combine with the resin of the balsam, thus forming a good binding excipient.

Copaiba was at one time ordered very frequently in pill form, and magnes. carb. levis was the favourite excipient, but the mass so made becomes as hard as stone and is not disintegrated in the alimentary canal. Probably a part of the volatile oil may be assimilated, but this is doubtful. A better plan is to make a gum emulsion of the 'balsam,' and then add 1 part of calcined magnesia to every 10 parts by weight of 'balsam.' In about twelve hours the emulsion should be of the consistence of a thick salve. Now, by the addition of a very small quantity of borax, a pill-mass is obtained which leaves nothing to be desired. A pill taken in the mouth is at once brought to the condition of an emulsion, and the mass will keep for a long time, only requiring when it is old to be worked up in a warm mortar. Phosphate of calcium is also a good excipient

Butyl-chloral Hydrate (Croton chloral) should not be treated with substances such as confection of hips or extract of gentian, which would give a dark-coloured mass. Whenever possible white substances should be made into white pills. Equal parts of powdered acacia, tragacanth, and syrup make good pills of croton chloral hydrate.

Calcium chloride.—Pills of this salt do not silver well unless special precautions be used. . Make a mass with Canada balsam. When rolled out and well rounded, coat the pills with tolu and ether, and after five minutes moisten them very slightly with thin mucilage, applied by the finger and thumb, drop them in the silver leaf, and proceed *secundum artem.* Send the pills out in a well-corked bottle, as they are likely to deliquesce.

Calomel.—A very good mass is made with manna. The following also makes an excellent pill :—

> Hydr. subchlor. . . . . . . gr. xxiv.
> Conf. rosæ canin. . . . . . . q.s.
> Pulv. tragac. . . . . . . gr. ij.
> M. Ft. pil. xij.

Camphor generally gives trouble, and is the rock upon which many candidates for examination are stranded. In the first place powder the camphor finely—it is preferable to use *flowers of camphor*—by the aid of a little spirit ; then, if the pill is to contain camphor simply, mass with glycerine of tragacanth. This also serves well for such a pill as—

> Ammonii carbonatis . . . . . gr. iss.
> Camphoræ . . . . gr. ss.

Some dispensers prefer to use soap and a little fixed oil for camphor alone, as in the following formulæ :—

> *Ordinary size Pills.*
>
> Camphor . . . . gr. xviij.
> Ol. olivæ . . . . gtt. iij.
> Saponis . . . . gr. iij.
> M. Ft. pil. vj.

Large size Pills.

Camphor .	. . . . . .	gr. xxiv.
Ol. ricini .	. . . . .	gtt. iij.
Saponis .	. . . . .	gr. ij.

M.   Ft. pil. vj.

When extract of henbane (or other green extract) is ordered along with camphor, powder the latter with the addition of a little water instead of spirit. The addition of the extract will then make a good plastic mass which retains its consistence for some time. If the extract should make the mass too soft, it may be stiffened with powdered curd soap, or a mixture of the same with liquorice.

When there is a large proportion of gum resin in a mass, rectified spirit is a good excipient, as in the following case :—

P. asafœtidæ	. . . . .	ʒv.
P. zinci oxidi	. . . . .	gr. xij.
P. camphoræ	. . . . .	gr. vj.
Ext. belladonnæ	. . . .	gr. iij.

Fiant pilulæ xxiv.

Another example :—

Ext. belladonnæ .	. . . .	gr. iv.
Pulv. camphoræ .	. . . .	ʒss.
Quininæ sulph. .	. . . .	ʒj.
Zinci sulph.	. . . .	gr. x.

M.   Ft. mas. et div. in pil. xxx.

In this case powder the camphor by aid of a drop or two of water and the zinc sulphate, add the quinine and extract, with a few grains of tragacanth, and make a softish mass with a mixture of 2 parts of simple syrup and 1 part of glycerine.

Carbolic Acid.—Absolute phenol in detached crystals is the most convenient form for the dispensing-counter, and especially for making pills. The excipients which are in use for carbolic acid number about half a dozen—viz. wheaten flour, powdered soap and liquorice, soap and tragacanth with glycerine, powdered althæa and a trace of glycerine, and one or two others. Success with either of these greatly depends upon habit ; the dispenser who is successful with soap and liquorice sticks to these as the best excipient, and so with others. The excipient to be used must depend greatly upon the nature of the mass. For example :—

Bismuthi subnitrat.	gr. iij.
Acid. carbol.	gr. j.
Fiat pil.	

This makes a good pill by rubbing up the acid with $\frac{1}{2}$ a grain of powdered curd soap, adding the subnitrate, and massing with a very little glycerine of tragacanth.

Another example:—

Podophylli resinæ	gr. $\frac{1}{6}$
Pil. rhei co.	gr. iij.
Acid. carbolic.	♏ j.
Fiat pil. j.	

Rub up the absolute phenol with an equal weight of soap ; then add the powdered ingredients of the rhubarb pill, the podophyllin, and a little powdered tragacanth. Mass with a little treacle.

Carbolic acid has very much the characteristics of creosote (which see).

Cascara Sagrada Extract.—Stiffen with tragacanth and liquorice and varnish the pills. Thus made they keep the shape perfectly.

Cinchonidine, and other cinchona alkaloids, may be treated as quinine (which see).

Corrosive Sublimate in pills should be first rubbed to a fine powder along with twice or three times its weight of sugar of milk, and the other ingredients, except the excipient, added little by little, so that a perfect mixture may be formed. Some authorities maintain that all potent substances should be combined in a state of solution, and the following form is given in illustration of this rule :—

Hydrarg. perchlor.	.	.	.	.	.	gr. j.
Glycerin.	.	.	.	.	.	gtt. j.
Conf. rosæ canin.	.	.	.	.	.	gr. v.
Pulv. acaciæ	.	.	.	.	.	gr. x.

M.   Ft. pil. viij.

The sublimate being dissolved in the glycerine, perfect distribution is effected. If the sublimate is dissolved in ether and the solution triturated with liquorice powder, the salt is obtained in a very finely divided state. Dzondi's sublimate pills are made with 0·75 gramme hydrarg. bichlor., with breadcrumb and sugar, each q.s. to make 250 pills. The salt should be thoroughly mixed with 3 grammes of sugar ; to this another 10 grammes of sugar should be added, 13 grammes of dried crumb, and 4·5 grammes of glycerinated water.

Creosote.—Mr. Martindale states that the best material for combining creosote into pills is powdered curd soap, B.P. Put the soap and the creosote in equal parts in a wide-mouthed stoppered bottle ; mix well, and digest in a water-bath till they combine. This, on cooling, forms a plastic mass suitable for forming pills, and can be combined with other ingredients, preferably in powder.

A few shreds of yellow wax, with a little powdered soap, when not incompatible, make good pills, but they are somewhat insoluble. Powdered liquorice may be substituted for the soap. Light calcined magnesia (1 grain to 2 minims of creosote) mixed with creosote solidifies in a few hours, and can then be easily worked into pills ; but this addition cannot be recommended, as the solubility of the pill is extremely doubtful. Mr. Martindale says that pills thus made are as insoluble as marbles. Always be careful about adding a chemical, such as magnesia : in most cases a chemical change is the result. Powdered soap, 1 part ; powdered liquorice-root, 5 parts : three grains of this mixture will make a good mass with 1 minim of creosote. Animal soap, it should be noted, is far better for massing pills than Castile soap. For example : Creosote gtt. xii., curd soap, dried and powdered, gr. vi., phosphate of lime q.s. This makes a good mass and a small pill, but with Castile soap this would not be the case.

Croton Oil.—Powdered curd soap, with a little glycerine of tragacanth, does well for croton oil. When a dispenser gets a prescription such as the following to dispense, the best plan is to add 2 grains of wheaten flour to each minim of oil, and mass with the confection :—

Ol. croton.	gtt. v.
Conf. rosæ	q.s.

Ft. pil. iv.

The dispenser who got this prescription melted 5 grains of yellow wax in a mortar and added the oil ; mixed and added 2 grains of confection, and massed with liquorice. It made a fair mass. But it is evident that such a procedure is very risky. Wax is a substance which is insoluble in aqueous fluids, and therefore in the alimentary canal ; if therefore it be added to pill-masses in such quantity that the *melting-point* of the mass is raised above the heat of the body, the pill will pass through the body unchanged.

Crystalline Salts, soluble in water, require a little care. They should be very finely powdered, and massed with thin conserve, adding, if necessary, a little tragacanth, or preferably with glycerine of tragacanth and a little inert powder. If silvered, they must be varnished with tolu, and allowed to dry, before using mucilage, or else silvered with the varnishing solution alone.

Potass. brom.	ℨss.
Ferri sulph.	ℨss.
Ext. nucis vom.	gr. ii.ss.
Ext. gentianæ .	q.s.

Fiant pilulæ xv.

In this formula double decomposition takes place between the two salts, the water of crystallisation in the sulphate of iron being liberated ; consequently, a very small quantity of extract suffices. Since bromide of iron is formed, the pills should be varnished and sent out in a bottle.

Quininæ sulph.	gr. xxiv.
Ferri sulph. exsic.	gr. xxiv.
Ferri arseniatis	gr. iss.
Ext. nucis vom.	gr. vj.
Ferri iodidi	gr. xlviij.

Fiant pilulæ xxiv. Varnish with tolu.

This is likely to prove troublesome. The iodide of iron (recently prepared) should be powdered in a warm mortar, the other ingredients added, together with 5 grains of glycerine of tragacanth ; the whole is to be vigorously worked together until it becomes plastic, rolled quickly, varnished, and enclosed in a bottle. Six or eight grains of extract of gentian also make a good mass.

Ergotin.—This is supplied of very varying consistence, some samples being quite thick and granular like extract of beef, others are smooth and semi-fluid. In either case it requires the addition of an inert vegetable powder, such as powdered althæa. If there be more than two grains in each pill it requires evaporation, in order to keep the pill of a reasonable size. The addition of about a twentieth part of tragacanth to each part of ergotin is an improvement.

Essential Oils.—The addition of wax or resin should be the last resort, but this is sometimes unavoidable, as in the following case, where the use of soap is objectionable owing to the double decomposition which would result between the ferrous sulphate and the soap :—

Ferri sulph. exsic.	gr. i⅕.
Ext. aloes aq.	gr. j.
Olei sabinæ	♏j.

M. Fiat pil. Mitte cxliv.

Melt 72 grains of yellow wax on a water-bath, and add the oil, gently beating if necessary till they are thoroughly mixed. Mix the aloes and ferrous sulphate with 12 grains of powdered tragacanth. Pour upon this the oil and wax. Mix well, and mass with a little glucose syrup. This makes a beautiful 4-grain pill.

Soap is generally all that is required to make a tractable mass—for example, a mixture of powdered soap, 1 part, and powdered liquorice-root, 5 parts. Three grains will make a good mass with 1 minim of an essential oil, and a little water or S.V.R. In such a case as the following the liquorice should of course be omitted :—

Pulv. rhei	gr. j.
Pulv. zingib.	gr. j.
Ol. carui	m j.

Misce. Fiat pilula.

Rub up the oil with 1 grain of powdered soap, add the powders and mass with the smallest possible quantity of treacle.

When the powders in a pill are resinous, as in ext. coloc. co., pil. asafœtid. co., aloes, etc., they should be triturated with the oil for a few minutes, the remaining ingredients, if any, added ; then, if too hard use S.V.R., or, if too soft, a sufficiency of liquorice and soap.

A little solution of potash is often of great service in a mass containing much essential oil. Its use, however, in the majority of cases is to be deprecated.

Essential oils frequently form good excipients, as in the following examples :—

Pil. hydrarg. . . .	gr. 4	Ext. nucis vom. . .	gr. ¼
P. ext. coloc. co. . .	gr. 6	Creosoti . . .	m j.
Podophyllin . . .	gr. ¼	Asafœtidæ . .	gr. iij.
Olei anthem. . .	m j.	P. glycyrrh. . .	gr. ij.
Fiant pilulæ ij.		Fiat pilula.	
P. pil. aloes et ferri .	ʒj.	Ext. hyoscy. . .	gr. j.
P. guaiaci res. . .	ʒj.	P. pil. coloc. co. .	gr. iv.
Ol. sabinæ . .	m xv.	Ol. cajeputi . .	m j.
Fiant pilulæ xxiv.		Fiat pilula.	

Ext. Cannabis Indicæ. — Liquorice or lycopodium makes a good mass ; failing which, equal parts of pulv. tragac. co. and carbonate of magnesia may be tried.

Extract Taraxaci.—A correspondent of *The Chemist and Druggist* had the following to dispense :—

Ext. nucis vom..	gr. iij.
Ext. tarax.	gr. xij.
Ext. aloes aq.	gr. iij.
Ext. hyoscy.	q.s.

M. Ft. pil. xii. (in arg.).

The pills split open after being silvered, even though varnished. The swelling in this case was no doubt due to the taraxacum extract, which is generally in a state of incipient decomposition, and silvered pills made of it frequently split. The best plan is to evaporate the extract almost to dryness and use a little tragacanth, as well as extract of henbane to mass. The mass should not be made too hard, and the pills should be allowed to stand for half an hour before silvering.

Fel Bovinum, with the addition of equal parts of tragacanth and acacia, forms good pills. The ox-gall may be bought in a dried and powdered state. In this condition it is very convenient, and forms an excellent mass with dec. aloes co. conc.

Ferri Bromidum.—The Société de Pharmacie de Paris recommends a hot strong solution of the bromide to be mixed in a dry warm porcelain mortar, with liquorice-powder and gum arabic in equal parts, sufficient to make a mass. The pills should be rolled in lycopodium or, better, coated with sugar, and preserved in a well-dried bottle. .

Ferri Iodidum.—Blancard's iodide of iron pills were formerly prescribed to be made as follows : Combine 4 grammes of iodine with 2 grammes of powdered iron in 8 grammes of water, filter upon 5 grammes of honey, evaporate to 10 grammes and make into pills with marshmallow and liquorice. A shorter and equally good process is to stir 2 grammes of iron with 4 grammes of iodine in 4 grammes of distilled water in a porcelain mortar until the brown colour has disappeared. Then mix 4 grammes white sugar, 3 grammes marshmallow, and 7·5 grammes liquorice. Make 100 pills, roll them in talc, and dry in a warm place. The dried pills to be varnished with balsam of tolu.

Ferri et Quininæ Citras.—For this many excipients are used, and success with any of them depends greatly on habit. Good pills, which keep their shape and do not deliquesce, can be made by using unguentum resinæ as an excipient. Both proof and rectified spirit make a good mass, but in both cases it must be rolled out quickly.

Ferri Sulphas.—The granulated sulphate should be used for pills; it is generally free from adhering moisture, can be readily reduced to impalpable powder and massed with glycerine of tragacanth with the addition of a little powdered sugar.

Ferri Sulph. Exsiccat. is a very variable compound as obtained from wholesale houses. Some samples, owing to over-heating, contain basic sulphate of iron. Dispensers should hesitate, therefore, before using the dried sulphate in place of the undried, in order to make a smaller pill. One peculiarity of the dried sulphate when in pills is that the pills are apt to crack.

Quin. sulph.	gr. xv.
Ext. bellad.	gr. x.
Ferri sulph. exsic.	ʒ j.

Fiant pil. xxx.

This was made into a mass with 4 grains of tragacanth and a little glycerine, but after about three weeks the pills cracked. A mixture of glycerine (1 part) and water (2 parts) makes a much better mass in this case, especially if a few grains of powdered acacia are used along with the tragacanth, and triturated with the iron salt before the other ingredients are added.

Ferruginous Pills (Blaud).—The original Blaud's pill was made by heating together sulphate of iron and carbonate of potash in honey, then adding other ingredients, and evaporating to a pilular consistence. The combination is now presented at the dispensing-counter in various forms, such as ferrous sulphate with carbonate of soda or potash. With these

we shall deal presently. First we may notice exceptional
methods of prescribing the pills, as the following :—

Ferri sulph. . . . . . . gr. ij.
Potas. bicarb. . . . . . gr. ij.
Confect. rosarum . . . . . q.s.
Ft. pil. tales cl.

Ferri sulph. granulat. . . . . gr. ijss.
Sodæ bicarb. . . . . . gr. ijss.
Glycerin. tragacanth . . . . q.s.
Ft. pil. Mitte xlviij.

Leaving out the question of massing in the meantime, it
will be noticed that sulphate of iron and an alkaline carbonate
or bicarbonate undergo double decomposition when brought
together. Thus, with a carbonate the reaction is according to
the following equation :—

$$FeSO_4, 7H_2O + Na_2CO_3 = FeCO_3 + Na_2SO_4 + 7H_2O.$$

With a bicarbonate it is as follows :—

$$FeSO_4, 7H_2O + 2NaHCO_3 = FeCO_3 + Na_2SO_4 + CO_2 + 8H_2O.$$

In the latter case the freed carbonic-acid gas greatly affects the
resulting mass. Either the salts must be allowed to lie until
all the gas is expelled (whereby the ferrous salt is much oxidised by exposure) and then massed ; or the mass may be made
right off, the consequence being that the pills are much larger
than they should be, owing to occluded gas. It is advisable,
therefore, in such cases as are quoted above, to substitute a
proportionate amount of the carbonate for the bicarbonate.

It is apparent also that, owing to the liberation of water of
crystallisation, soft excipients, such as are given in the above
prescriptions, are inapplicable.

Opinions regarding Blaud's pills are very varied. Whitla,
for example, considers that when a prescription is received for
pills containing $2\frac{1}{2}$ gr. of sulphate of iron and $2\frac{1}{2}$ gr. of carbonate of potash, a mass should be made with a little vaseline and
cacao-butter in order to avoid decomposition. A *Chemist and
Druggist* annotator, evidently of a similar school, says : 'It is

desirable to form a mass in which the minimum of chemical action takes place during the massing. For this purpose, the salts are each reduced to powder separately, then intimately mixed with a twelfth of their combined weight of tragacanth, and made into a mass with a twentieth of their weight of water.'

Hager advises to rub the iron salt in an iron mortar with the alkaline carbonate until a damp mass is formed, which is set aside for fifteen or twenty minutes. It is then of a thin muddy consistence. To this is added about three-tenths of its weight of tragacanth and a few drops of glycerinated water, and the mass is set aside for another ten minutes. If it is then at all crumbly, a few more drops of glycerinated water may be added, and a good mass will be formed.

It is not advisable to follow either of these methods at the dispensing-counter. Mix the salts together, add a twentieth of their weight of powdered tragacanth and the same of sugar, and mass quickly with as little water as possible, about 5 minims sufficing for a dozen 5-grain pills. It should be noted that equal proportions of the alkaline carbonate and ferrous sulphate give an excess of the alkali. Three parts of carbonate of potash and 5 of sulphate of iron are better proportions. The following is the B.P.C. formula :—

Sulphate of iron	60 grains
Carbonate of potassium	36 ,,
Sugar, in powder	12 ,,
Tragacanth, in powder	4 ,,
Glycerine	2½ minims
Distilled water	a sufficient quantity

Reduce the sulphate of iron to fine powder, add the sugar and tragacanth, and mix intimately. Finely powder the carbonate of potassium in another mortar, and thoroughly incorporate with it the glycerine. Transfer this to the mortar containing the sulphate of iron, beat thoroughly until the mass becomes green, and add water sufficient to impart a soft pilular consistence, and divide into twenty-four pills.

Each pill contains about 1 grain of ferrous carbonate.

Ferrum Redactum should be rubbed down to fine powder, a little liquorice added, and a mass made with glycerine of tragacanth ; or manna alone may be used. When combined with vegetable extracts containing, as most do, some acid ingredients, the addition of any moisture, according to Hager, occasions the development of hydrogen and combination of the iron, the pills being liable to swell. Of course, the extracts should not be acid.

Guaiacate of Lithia.—Powder finely, and use proof spirit, ℥ viij. to ʒj. ; a *soft* mass should be made, and slight warmth will be found of advantage.

Hydrargyrum c. Cretâ must not be vigorously worked in the pill-mortar, or mercury separates ; thin conserve or a soft extract forms a good excipient. If prescribed with powders or pill-masses which can be used in powder, grey powder should be carefully triturated with such ingredients first ; there is then little chance of mercury being separated. For instance—

Hydrarg. c. cretâ .	.	.	.	.	.	gr. iij.
Ext. hyoscy. .	.	.	.	.	.	gr. iij.
Pulv. pil. coloc. co.	.	.	.	.	.	gr. iij.

Fiant pilulæ ij.

Insoluble Salts.—For substances insoluble, or nearly so, in water, and entirely devoid of adhesive property, such as oxysalts of bismuth, oxalate of cerium, etc., the glycerine of tragacanth is one of the best excipients. In some cases a mixture of equal parts acacia and tragacanth and syrup give more adhesiveness and excellent results.

Lupulin and Camphor are not readily made into a plastic mass by the usual excipients without considerably increasing the size of the pills, but ether very sparingly used yields a good mass without any other addition.

Pepsin.—Make a rather soft mass with a mixture of equal parts of glycerine, syrup, and water, and roll quickly. Five grains of pepsin and acid. hydrochlor. dil. ℥ j make a very good mass.

Phosphorus.— The phosphorus pill of the Pharmacopœia has never become a favourite, because, as first introduced, the mass was so hard as to be perfectly insoluble in the alimentary canal. The formula has now been improved. Mr. A. C. Abraham has recommended a mass made simply with balsam of tolu. He points out, however, that the balsam must be washed in order to free it from several bodies lighter than water, and to remove certain contaminations such as cinnamic and benzoic acid. Moreover, the resinous matter is thus satu-rated with as much water as it is capable of retaining. The mass is made as follows :—

Washed balsam of tolu	960 grains
Phosphorus, pure	40 ,,

Place the tolu and phosphorus in a suitable enamelled iron basin, capable of holding about 40 oz. and containing about 20 oz. of water. Heat the basin in a water-bath, and when the ingredients are thoroughly melted stir with a glass rod until particles of phosphorus can no longer be seen, taking care that the ingredients are not brought above the surface of the water. Continue the stirring constantly for fifteen minutes, remove the basin from the water-bath, place it under a tap, and pour over it cold water. When sufficiently cool, mix it further under the water with the hands for a short time, and finally place it under water in earthenware jars.

One grain of this mass contains $\frac{1}{25}$ of a grain of phosphorus divided into 10,000 particles! The mass may be combined with any other ingredients. Phosphorus pills made with cacao-butter as the only excipient dissolve so readily that the phosphorus causes unpleasant eructations, but a smaller dose given in this way appears to be more effective.

Messrs. Allen & Hanburys, some years since, published the following formula for *Pil. phosphori cum sapone,* and it has become a great favourite with pharmacists :—

Phosphori . . . . . gr. ij.
Carbon. bisulph. . . . ♏x. vel q.s.
Solve.

Pulv. saponis dur. . . . gr. xxxv.
Pulv. guaiaci resin. . . . gr. xxxv.
Glycerin. . . . . gtt. xij.-
Pulv. rad. glycyrrh. . . . gr. xij, vel q.s.

Ut fiat massa gr. c. To be divided into pills of the strength required, and varnished or coated in the ordinary way.

The mass is of good consistence, easily manipulated, and readily soluble. A drop of oil of cloves added to the carbon bisulphide is said by Mr. Proctor to lessen its tendency to inflame.

The bisulphide of carbon method is the most expeditious for the dispensing-counter. The method which is generally most successful is to rub up some liquorice-powder ($\frac{1}{2}$ to 1 grain for each pill) with half its weight of water, pour on the bisulphide solution, stir well and without pressure, and make into a mass with compound tragacanth powder. The water effectually prevents oxidation of the phosphorus, and the bisulphide is dissipated in massing.

This method is also suitable in such a case as the following :—

Quininae sulphatis . . . . gr. $\frac{1}{2}$
Ext. nucis vom. . . . . gr. $\frac{1}{4}$
Phosphori . . . . . gr. $\frac{1}{33}$

If you have to make, say, 33 pills, rub the quinine and extract together with 15 grains of powdered liquorice and 5 drops of water. Now dissolve the phosphorus in 5 or 6 drops of bisulphide of carbon in a small test-tube ; mix with the other ingredients, and mass quickly with glycerine of tragacanth. Phosphorus pills should always be varnished or coated with a solution of wax in ether (1 in 7), and finished off with French chalk.

Pil. Aloes et Myrrhæ.—The best excipient is a mixture of glycerine 1 part, and treacle 3 parts.

Pil. Coloc. Co. as now made with resin of scammony invariably flattens. This is prevented to some extent by adding from ten to twenty drops of potash solution to the ounce of mass or by substituting soap for the sulphate of potash. The addition of a fibrous powder such as liquorice gives durability to the mass. Pil. coloc. c. hyos. requires only the extract to mass it.

Pil. Hydrargyri.—When this is prescribed with a soft extract the latter should, if possible, be dried or used in powder.

Pil. Hydrarg. Subchlor. Co., with pill-masses having an aqueous excipient, invariably forms a crumbly combination; this is remedied by using the former in powder—*i.e.* by omitting the castor-oil.

Potassii Iodidum may be made into pills, according to Whitla, by rubbing the salt with a few drops of water into a stiff smooth paste, and working it into a good mass by the addition of a little liquorice-powder; in this way 6 grains may be easily got into a fair-sized pill. Tragacanth and water alone make a good mass.

A pill containing this iodide and a considerable quantity of extract of colchicum was ordered, and although carefully dried extract was used, the mass proved to be too soft. As the pills were not required till next day they were placed under a bell jar (really a mortar upside down), with sulphuric acid. This proved a success, and has often been found useful with an otherwise refractory pill.

Potassii Permanganas.—Some years ago the proposal to administer this highly oxidising compound in pill form for certain female complaints brought out a number of suggestions as to the manner in which the permanganate should be made into pill. Obviously no substance which is readily oxidised, such as extract of gentian or glycerine of tragacanth amongst common pill excipients, should be used. The excipient must be a substance which is practically unoxidisable, and such

we have in various fats and earths. For example, resin ointment 1 part, and permanganate of potash 4 parts, make a good
mass, but if kept for some time it disintegrates with great difficulty. Mr. Martindale at first used vaseline, then a mixture of
vaseline and paraffin, but the mass wanted firmness ; then he
added kaolin, which gave it the desired firmness.

The mixture under the name of *kaolin ointment* is now a
regular stock excipient. It contains equal parts of paraffin,
vaseline, and kaolin. The fats are melted and the kaolin sifted
into the mixture while hot, and constantly stirred till cold. A
very good mass is also made with kaolin and water, or with
fuller's earth and water. Mr. Proctor, of Newcastle, strongly
advocated the kaolin 'without grease' in preference to Mr.
Martindale's excipient ; 18 grains of powdered fuller's earth
and 12 grains of permanganate of potash make a good mass
with a little water. Mr. Martindale recommends the pills to
be coated with sandarach varnish, but this is questionable
advice, for the alcohol penetrates the pill, and is oxidized by a
portion of the permanganate. It is better to give the pills a
thin coating with a solution of white wax or paraffin in benzene,
afterwards finishing off with French chalk.

The following prescription has to be treated on the principles laid down in the foregoing :—

Ferri mangan. . . . . 3j.
Ferri oxyd. . . . . 3j.
Cinchonin. mur. . . . . . . 3iss.
Ft. pil. 48. Silver.

Make a mixture of paraffin and vaseline, of each half a drachm,
and to this add the cinchonidine previously rubbed down fine,
then add the manganate and oxide of iron, both in fine powder,
and stiffen with a little kaolin if necessary.

Quinine Sulphate.—The simplest excipient is glycerine
of tragacanth, or five per cent. of tragacanth well mixed forms
a very good mass with simple syrup ; a *little* glycerine may
be added if the pills are to be kept long. The use of extract
of gentian or other dark-coloured excipients is objectionable,

as it is now universally recognised that white substances should be formed into white pill-masses. For this reason sulphuric acid alone is now extensively used as an excipient, 1 drop being sufficient for 4 grains of quinine ; mass quickly and roll in French chalk or fine sifted arrowroot.

An excellent mass is made with tartaric acid and a little glycerine and water. For a dozen 5-grain pills take 6 grains of tartaric acid and rub it up with the quinine until it becomes crumbly, then add two drops each of glycerine and water, and mass quickly. Some object to tartaric acid because it alters the chemical constitution of the quinine salt, sulphotartrate being formed, but this is therapeutically the same as the sulphate.

The dispenser must use his judgment as to what may be the best excipient in unusual cases ; for example, with such a prescription as the following :—

Quin. sulph.	gr. iss.
Picis liquid.	gr. iij.
M. Ft. pil. j., sec. art. mitte xx., j. ter. die.	

In this case an inert powder, such as lycopodium or liquorice, adds too greatly to the bulk of the pill. If melted with a fifth of its weight of wax, the tar becomes more tractable, and masses well with calcium phosphate.

Resinous Ingredients in Pills.—Gum resins and resins must be first rubbed to a fine powder, and, to prevent them sticking to the mortar, the latter and the pestle may be first rubbed with paper soaked in almond oil. The resinous powder is easily made into a mass with a few drops of spirit, but the pills so made do not keep their shape. To most of such substances, to aloes especially, the addition of a little vegetable powder or scraped blotting-paper is desirable. Asafœtida gives pills of good consistence with a few drops of weak spirit ; but such an addition with aloes produces pills which flatten. Spirit should be added very cautiously, as it is often found, especially when any soap is present, that on working the mass becomes softer than it at first appears. Mucilage of acacia is, according to a contributor, a much safer excipient than spirit.

If spirit is used the main thing to be observed is not to add too much of it. The mass, for example, should never be made so soft as those made with ordinary excipients, but should on the contrary be so hard as to roll only with some degree of pressure. If this be attended to they will not fall. Where, however, the pills require to be kept for a length of time, some less drying excipient should be used. In all cases where pills are composed mainly of resins, too much friction with the rounder in finishing them should be avoided. We have had occasion frequently to observe the peculiar effect which sharp friction (probably from the heat developed) produces on various resinous substances in the way of changing their physical properties, and in many cases the principal cause of pills falling is due as much to the friction used in rounding them with the finisher as to the excipient used.

Rhei Pulvis.—Use proof spirit or tincture of rhubarb ($\mathfrak{m}$ j. to 3 gr.); a *soft* mass should be made and rolled quickly, otherwise it is troublesome. Only 24 pills should be made at once, or the mass assumes a leathery condition, and has to be thrown away.

Pulv. rhei .	. . , ...	3j.
P. saponis dur. .	. . . . . .	3j.
Pulv. ipecac.	. . . , . . .	gr. vj.
Fiant pilulæ xxiv.		

This makes a good mass with tincturæ rhei $\mathfrak{m}$ xxv.

Rhubarb is, like many other substances, one for which each dispenser has his own excipient, as may be judged from the following given by skilled pharmacists :—

(1) Simple syrup is better than either spirit or water for massing powdered rhubarb.

(2) Use a mixture of equal parts glycerine and tincture of rhubarb ($\mathfrak{m}$ j. to 3 grs.).

(3) For powdered rhubarb, a mixture of glycerine two parts, rectified spirit one part, answers well.

(4) Powdered rhubarb makes a good mass with one-fifth its weight of glycerine.

(5) Treacle is the most valuable excipient for powdered rhubarb.

Sodæ Bicarb.—Three grains of dry bicarbonate of soda with 1 grain of powdered ginger can be made into a very workable mass by the addition of 1 grain of tragacanth, and water or mucilage sufficient to make a mass. The pills both roll well and keep well.

Sulphide of Calcium, now much ordered in minute doses for acne, should be mixed with an equal quantity of sugar of milk, and, after careful trituration, as much powdered decorticated liquorice-root added as will make the weight up to, say, a grain. The mass can now be easily worked up with a little glycerine of tragacanth.

Tannic Acid.—If these pills be made with mucilage they, as soon as dry, crack, crumble, and fall to powder. A mixture of glycerine and mucilage of acacia makes an excellent excipient.

Zinci Valer.—Add a small quantity of acacia, and mass with spirit. This gives a mass requiring quick manipulation, but yielding excellent results. Glycerine of tragacanth also makes a good mass with the addition of a little inert vegetable powder.

EXCIPIENTS.

Acacia Powder by itself is an excipient of very little value for the purpose of giving consistence; but, with the addition of 10 per cent. of pulv. althææ, it becomes, according to Hager, a good excipient, helping to form a mass of good consistence, which binds well.

Bread-crumb is stated to be an excellent excipient for many things, but it is curious that it is rare to find anyone who uses it. Some time back in the present century it was recommended to the apprentice as a good excipient for making creosote into pills; carbolic acid was not discovered, or that would have been included in his instructions. It is mournful to reflect how popular fallacies get perpetuated. Having tried this excipient under all the forms indicated in text-books, and witnessed many repeating the experiment, we may fairly assert that in every case an equal, if not a better, excipient could have been employed. Either the mass crumbles, or is in an unmanageable paste, or oozes with uncombined oily matter. Pills *can* be made with bread-crumb, but they require such attention, and so frequently disappoint the dispenser, that the excipient is not worthy to retain a place in practical pharmacy. When 'mica panis' is ordered as an excipient, use wheat-flour and water q.s., if these will make a mass with the medicinal ingredients.

Calcii Phosphas possesses in a very remarkable degree the property of giving a greasy substance, such as lard or mercurial ointment, a good pilular consistence, when added in comparatively small quantity.

Confection of Roses and **Confection of Hips** increase the bulk of pills more than is liked nowadays.

Decoctum Aloes Co. is sometimes useful where a considerable quantity of oil has to be combined with a rather soft mass. It is an excellent excipient for most pills containing aloes, but is to be avoided where the carbonate of potassium contained in it would prove an incompatible.

Extract of Malt is a capital excipient for general use.

Glucose (or **Honey**) is a serviceable excipient in many cases.

Glycerine keeps pills soft, but, being a very hygroscopic body itself, it cannot be used with other hygroscopic bodies. Glycerine ceases to show this character when it contains at least one-third of its weight of moisture. Whenever glycerine alone has been used, add about 1 to 2 grains, as the case requires, of tragacanth. Add the gum *after* the action of the glycerine has taken place, not simultaneously. The observation which has been made that glycerine ceases to be hygroscopic when mixed with non-hygroscopic powders is not borne out by our experience. On keeping such pill-masses for a given time, we find the contrary. There is a risk, at all events, of deliquescent action. Glycerine 1 part, with treacle 3 parts, is an excellent excipient for pil. aloes et myrrhæ. Manna and glycerine are very useful as an excipient in many cases—for example, in making nitrate of silver or calomel pills.

Mucilage of Acacia as an excipient should be avoided. It makes pills too hard ; indeed, with some substances (such as calomel) it forms a perfect cement.

Pulv. Althææ, if used largely, has a tendency, in consequence of its large proportion of mucilage, to interfere with the solubility of the pills, and to reduce their activity. Besides, it is apt to make the mass too elastic to work well into shape, and to harden too much afterwards. Not more than 1 grain to 5 or 10 grains should be used. Three parts of marshmallow powder require 2 parts of water to form a mass. Hager states that in large German dispensing businesses the following powders are sometimes kept ready for pills that require a binding excipient :—

For White Pills.		For Coloured Pills.	
Pulv. althææ . . . 10		Pulv. althææ . . . 15	
Farinæ secalinæ . . . 10		Farinæ secalinæ . . . 10	
Sacch. alb. 10		·Sacch. alb. 10	
Pulv. iridis 70		Pulv. iridis 50	
M. Ft. pulv. subtil.		Pulv. gentianæ . . . 15	
		M. Ft. pulv. subtil.	

Soap-powder makes the best pill-mass with vegetable powders, extracts, and gum resins. Soap being decomposed by acid salts, acids, many metallic salts and tannin substances, it is not suitable for masses containing these. In using soap care must be taken not to add too much water. Soap-masses at first appear dry and crumbly, so that the dispenser is tempted to add more water, and then finds afterwards that he has too soft a mass. A little spirit has this effect to a still greater extent, so that it must be used very carefully. Powdered curd soap is better than hard olive oil soap.

Spirit should not be used when there is much resin in the pill, and pills made with it should be rolled off very quickly, or they will crumble.

Sugar without some mucilaginous addition is not good. Syrup, however, with pulv. althææ is very useful.

Theriacanth.—A correspondent writes : 'For some months past during daily work at the dispensing-counter I have found a compound of treacle and tragacanth to be an excellent excipient, especially in pills requiring an adhesive excipient, such as ferrum redactum. For the sake of a name it was termed " theriacanth," and is made thus : Rub 1 drachm of pulv. tragacanth with 2 drachms of rectified spirit in a mortar ; then add quickly 2 oz. of treacle (previously made more fluid by warming), and thoroughly mix. This composition soon sets into an adhesive mass.'

Tragacanth gives solidity and elasticity to a mass a little too soft, but if too much be added the pills become so elastic that it is almost impossible to round them with the finisher. Tragacanth is especially to be recommended when the mass is too soft, and when it is desired not too much to increase the weight. If masses crumble, a little tragacanth-powder, with a few drops of glycerine, will bind them.

The objection to it on the ground of the subsequent cracking of the pill is without foundation, and the cause must be looked for elsewhere; frequently it results from some decomposition or reaction between the substances of the mass. The following is a good example, communicated by a correspondent of *The Chemist and Druggist*. He made a batch of Blaud's pills. First he mixed the sulphate of iron with the carbonate of potash, then added some sugar of milk and let stand in the mortar until thoroughly moist, then added tragacanth, and let the mass stand till it was getting firm, then weighed and rolled out. The pills thus made were left in a wooden tray exposed to the air for a few days, subsequently a 2-oz. wide-mouth bottle was filled with them and corked. The pills thus kept split; those kept in the tray exposed to the air did not. We received a sample of the pills. Those which had been kept in a bottle were quite crumbly, and few crystals of sulphate of iron were observable in them. Those kept in air were, on the other hand, hard and full of crystals of the sulphate, so that it would appear that in the former case the reaction between the sulphate of iron and carbonate of potash had gone further than in the latter case, and therefore that more ferrous carbonate had been formed. The formation of ferrous carbonate is accompanied by liberation of water, which uniting with the tragacanth would cause the pills to swell. The appearance of the coating of the pills which had been kept in a tray corroborated this, for it had become of a light brown colour, due to the united action of ferric iron and evaporating water, whereas the others were almost white.

Tragacanth (Glycerine of).—Nothing yet has proved of such general usefulness as this invention of Mr. Barnard

Proctor. His formula is now official. The gelatinous mass is binding, non-hygroscopic, and may be used with advantage in an infinite variety of everyday dispensing. It is still the dispenser's favourite in England, and is the best excipient for salts and metallic oxides, such as potassium bromide and bismuth subnitrate. The mass should be well kneaded, or more of the excipient will be used than is really necessary. For some other substances the official preparation is too thick and tough, but this may be remedied by the cautious addition of a little glycerine and water to the pill ingredients.

Tragacanth (Compound Powder).—This is useful in many cases. It is absorbing, binding, and preservative.

Unguentum Resinæ makes good pills of ferri et quininæ citras.

Water and Spirit as Excipients.—Many substances do not require the addition of an adhesive excipient—*e.g.* the extracts of aloes, pulv. pil. coloc. co., p. ext. coloc. co., etc., form a good mass with water (about ♏ iv. to ʒj.) ; p. pil. asafœt. co. is readily massed with rectified spirit. Pil. aloes et ferri gets exceedingly hard in a short time, and should be kept in powder, omitting the confection, and adding ½ oz. of liquorice to the B.P. quantities ; then 2 of the powder = 3 of the mass.

Wax in small shavings, with a little powdered soap where not incompatible, was at one time the recognised excipient for essential oils, carbolic acid, creosote, etc., but, as previously explained, there are objections to its use.

PRECAUTIONS.

In the original treatise Mr. Joseph Ince, Lecturer on Pharmacy to the Pharmaceutical Society, wrote regarding the use and abuse of some excipients ; and from his remarks we extract the following paragraphs :—

Excipients to be avoided are—(1) Those incompatible with any of the ingredients of the pill-mass. Thus, confection of roses must not be used to make up iron compounds ; acetic extract of colchicum must not be stiffened with magnesia. (2) Those which make the pills either too hard or too soft. (3) Those which unduly increase size.

Cera Flava will bind any coloured essential oil into a convenient mass ; while **Cera Alba** is used with the colourless ol. terebinth. Wax has come into some disfavour for internal use. It is effectual as an excipient, but not a necessity.

Decoct. Aloes Comp. is invaluable as an excipient for pills containing aloes and gum resins. Wonderfully small quantities are required, and it is not only effective, but a brilliant, glossy appearance is communicated. Where soap is also present still smaller quantities must be employed.

Liquor Potassæ has deservedly gone out of repute. Its convenience is undoubted, but its chemical action is regarded with suspicion. Pills so made frequently become tough, but this is not invariable.

Ol. Ricini, with or without soap, forms a good excipient for camphor pills.

Pulv. Tragac. Simpl.—In sparing quantities, and employed with discretion, there is no more serviceable excipient. The chief caution is to allow time, for it is surprising how small quantities will prove effective. Let the chemical action take place first ; warm gently ; then, and not before, add tragacanth. Attention to this remark will be of service to the manipulator, and many otherwise hopeless masses may so be reduced. Take this difficult formula as an illustration :—

Camphor	.	.	.	.	.	.	gr. vj.
Pil. galban. comp.	.	.	.	.	.	gr. xviij.
Ext. cannabis ind.	.	.	.	.	.	gr. iij.
Pulv. tragac.	.	.	.	.	.	gr. iij. (only)

M. Ft. pil. vj.

Let the camphor and Indian hemp deliquesce ; add the galbanum, previously warmed gently ; when the inevitable action has taken place add 3 grains of powdered tragacanth.

Water alone may be used as an excipient, as in opium pills, but the use of water needs a very practised hand to make it successful. The mass may be as soft as paste or hard as flint. 'In medio tutissimus ibis.' Water is introduced here in order to draw the attention of an inexperienced dispenser to one point. Its real use is by partial solution of the ingredients to diminish bulk, after which add the proper excipient. One drop of water or one drop of glycerine will often effect wonders in this way, and pills that otherwise would be of inconvenient size can be most elegantly dispensed.

Spirit Vini Rect., from its volatility and the subsequent hardness of the pills, may also be discarded.

We may conveniently sum up this chapter with some remarks by

MR. A. W. GERRARD ON PILL-MAKING.

What are the conditions required of a well-made pill? (1) The ingredients of which it is composed should be worked into an intimate admixture, no individual particles being discernible. (2) The parts should be held together by some cohesive force, sufficient to withstand the process of rolling and cutting without undergoing crumbling or cracking. (3) The pills being formed should retain under ordinary conditions a perfectly globular form. (4) The excipient, whether indicated by the prescriber or left to the discretion of the dispenser, should be chemically and therapeutically compatible with the other ingredients. (5) The pills should disintegrate readily soon after ingestion.

Failure to produce the preceding conditions may be ascribed to a variety of causes, as, for example : Excess or deficiency of a moist extract; presence of hygroscopic or deliquescent bodies; chemical incompatibility of ingredients; excess of essential or fixed oils; injudicious choice and use of excipients; bad manipulation.

The following are some prescriptions illustrating cases of failure, and the means of overcoming them :—

Ext. nucis vom. . . . . . . gr. $\frac{1}{3}$
  ,, hyoscy . . . . . . gr. iij.
Pulv. ipecac. . . . . gr. $\frac{1}{2}$
Fiat pilula.

Pills made from these ingredients soon lose their round form, becoming moist and unsightly ; the addition of $\frac{1}{2}$ grain of tragacanth powder sets all right, by absorbing moisture and imparting solidity.

Ext. colch. acet. . . . . . . gr. $\frac{1}{3}$
  ,, hyoscy. . . . . gr. iij.
Pil. hydrarg. . . . . gr. ij.
Fiat pil. Mane et nocte sumend.

This pill has the same defects as the previous one, but the material of each pill, $5\frac{1}{2}$ grains, makes it too .bulky to risk an addition. The difficulty can be got over by drying the extract of henbane on a pill-tile over a water-bath. Bear in mind volatile bodies must not be so treated.

Argenti oxidi . . . . gr. ij.
Pil. rhei co. . . . . gr. iij.
Fiat pil. Sumend. ante cibum.

Of all masses I think this is the most obstinate and vexing, becoming rapidly tough and unmanageable, the result of incompatibility, the silver salt being slowly reduced. A small admixture of confection of hips with the oxide at starting generally gives a good result.

Ol. caryoph. . . . . ♏ j.
Ext. col. co. . . . . gr. ij.
  ,, anthem. . . . . gr. ij.
Fiat pil.

Here essential oil is in excess, and the ingredients refuse to form a tenacious mass. In such a case the addition of $\frac{1}{2}$ grain of soap per pill brings them under control. Soap should not be used for salts of iron, lead, bismuth, copper, or mercury, as oleates would be formed.

Olei crotonis . . . . ♏ j.
Fiat pilula statim.

For this pill crumb of bread is often used as an excipient, but is a bad one, the pills on rolling having a troublesome elasticity, making it difficult to get them round. Nothing is better, in my experience, than 2 grains of compound tragacanth powder and 1 grain of soap for each pill. This excipient subdues croton oil most perfectly, and is equally suitable for creosote and carbolic acid.

Compound tragacanth powder is about the best general pill excipient. The simplicity of its constituents admirably adapts it as a diluent of all substances given in small doses ; whilst under its influence, in the presence of a little water, the most obstinate ingredients are brought under control. Solubility with easy disintegration is another of its characteristics. When oils have to be dealt with, a little soap may be added to the tragacanth with advantage.

COATING PILLS.

GILDING AND SILVERING.

COVERING pills with gold or silver leaf is a process which need not be described at great length. Silvering has largely gone out of fashion, and gilding is a refinement of pharmacy which the chemist is rarely called upon to perform. Like all pills which are to be coated, those that are to be silvered should be of firm consistence, and no powder should be used in rolling them out.

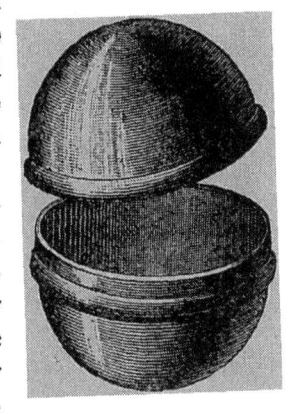

Pills containing asafœtida, and especially those containing sulphur or sulphides, should be very stiff, otherwise the metal will blacken after a few days. It is preferable to varnish the pills in this case. A covered pot may be used to silver the pills, but the box-wood silverer represented in the above cut is generally employed.

If the pills have been varnished with tolu, it may be necessary to moisten them with weak potash solution, instead of mucilage, as the latter will not always adhere to the resinous surface. One leaf of silver covers six 5-grain pills. One drop of weak mucilage is sufficient to damp a dozen such pills, and they should have a dull, not a glistening, appearance when thrown on the silver. The wetter the pills are the more silver-leaf is required, and the finish is not so good.

G

Sugar Coating.

This kind of coating has become popular, but the operation is somewhat difficult to perform on a small scale. Dr. Symes states that by practice it may be successfully carried out by the following process : Pills well dried on the surface are placed in a tinned copper bowl, such as is represented in the illus-

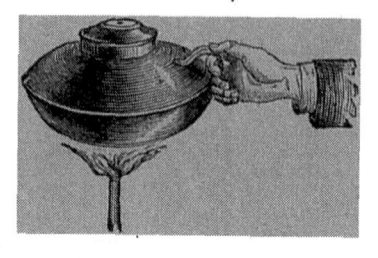

tration, with a flat bottom, or an enamelled iron dish, the surface of which has been moistened with syrup, or syrup and gum. They are then rotated and gently heated, very finely powdered sugar being dusted on, and the motion kept up till a perfectly dry, hard, and whitish coating is obtained, the operation being repeated if necessary. The first attempt is generally a failure, but practice is the only secret.

The following methods have also been proposed :—

Albumen and Sugar.—Pills sufficiently firm and dry should be rolled between the finger and thumb with enough white of egg to give them a thin coating. They should then be placed with finely powdered white sugar in a suitable vessel and rotated. The coating looks well and has a pleasant taste.

French Chalk and Sugar.—The pills are moistened with syrup or mucilage, or a mixture of the two, by shaking in a covered pot. They are then transferred to a box containing powdered French chalk or a mixture of French chalk and sugar, and are well shaken, and again transferred to a warm pill-tray and kept rapidly rotating until dry and smooth. The operation takes but little time.

The dispenser should not, however, expect to turn out pills with a sugar coating so elegant in appearance as that which is exhibited by commercial sugar-coated pills. These are coated by machinery (confectioner's revolving pans), the coating solution being a mixture of syrup and starch.

PEARL COATING.

A form of coating pills which has become popular in recent years is known as pearl coating. The powder used in this case is generally plain French chalk, or a mixture of French chalk with fine powdered sugar. In pearl coating, as also in sugar coating and silver coating, the following points must be attended to to ensure success—namely, the pills must be sufficiently dry and hard to prevent interstitial moisture exuding, and so spoiling the coating; they must be evenly but not excessively damped with thin mucilage; and, lastly, they must be thoroughly rotated, first in the powder and afterwards without any free powder, to produce a brilliant surface.

Very full particulars are given in the 'Art of Pharmacy' for coating pills for stock. The process there described is suitable for use at the dispensing-counter. The apparatus which is employed is after the pattern of the ordinary boxwood silverer, and is simply a tin globe copper-lined, about $5\frac{1}{2}$ inches diameter, intersected in the middle, the two sections being fixed with two brass pins. This arrangement permits of the apparatus being easily taken apart and thoroughly cleansed. In practice, two globes are generally sufficient, namely, one to coat and one to burnish the pills; but if a very high finish is required, a third will be necessary to polish the pills. This is done by thinly coating the warmed globe with white wax. The pills, after passing the second globe, are transferred to the waxed globe, and slowly rotated for a time in it. This gives them a brighter, more uniform, and probably, also, a more permanent coating.

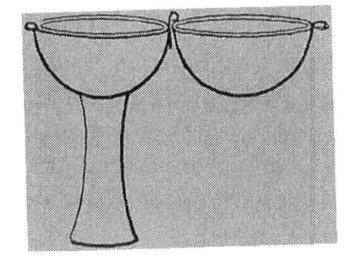

Take 1 drachm mucilage of acacia, and 1 drachm simple syrup, and add water sufficient to make 1 oz. Of this mixture pour sufficient upon the pills to damp the surface thoroughly

—the exact quantity can only be determined by experience— and after rotating in the coater in order to distribute the gum-mixture uniformly over the surface, add French chalk in *very fine powder*, and rotate uniformly until the chalk has all been taken up, or the pills thoroughly coated. If too little chalk has been used, or too much mucilage, more chalk will have to be added from time to time until the coating is uniform, at which point the pills may be transferred to the burnisher.

The following is another process which has been specially recommended for use at the dispensing-counter. It turns out a perfectly finished pearl-coated pill in a few minutes. Shake the pills in a covered pot with sandarach and ether varnish and throw into very fine French chalk, rotate for a minute, and separate excess of powder. Shake the pills in another pot with a mixture of equal parts of whipped white of egg (strained), syrup, and water, sufficient to thoroughly wet the pills, and throw them into excess of *very fine* French chalk, shake for a minute, remove the pills to a flat marble slab, and rotate *very lightly* under a pill-finisher, sprinkling on a very little chalk until a smooth surface is produced. If time permits they should be exposed to the air in a tray to dry thoroughly.

Martindale recommends *three* covered pots to be used. His moistening solution is composed of tragacanth 4 gr., syrup ʒss., water to ℥i.

Gelatine Coating.

Recent observations have shown that the gelatine coating is the most soluble of all. Apart from that, it has two important advantages. In the first place, the coating is transparent, so that the colour of the pill may be observed, and this in many cases is useful. Secondly, the coating is more quickly imparted than any other.

Thompson's gelatine pill-coating machine, illustrated and described in the 'Art of Pharmacy,' is specially applicable to coating large quantities. We have used the following simple device, in the absence of a better, with good results. If, say, three dozen pills are to be coated, take three soda-water corks, and stick into one end of each the eye-ends of a dozen needles at an angle of 45° ; then place a pill on each of the needles. The pills are now ready to receive the coating. An excellent solution is made from the following formula :—

French gelatine	. . . . . .	4 oz.
Gum acacia	. . . . . ; .	1 ,,
Boric acid	. . . .	2 dr.
Water	. . . .	40 oz.

Macerate the gelatine and acacia in the water for twelve hours, and dissolve by heating in water-bath. Add the boric acid, and strain through muslin.

A quantity of this may be made and stocked, and when required sufficient of it should be melted over a water-bath and kept liquid while being used. Dip the 'corkful' of pills into the solution, withdraw, and allow the drops of superfluous gelatine to form ; these may be removed by touching the surface of the liquid, then twirl the cork between the forefingers for a few seconds, and set aside to harden.

Varnishing Pills.

A very useful varnish is that made from tolu syrup residues by dissolving in ether. One ounce of the resinous residue in 3 oz. methylated ether is a suitable strength. This solution when applied to the pills evaporates rapidly. Martindale recommends a solution of sandarach 1 part in 1 of absolute alcohol. Hager recommends 5 parts of powdered mastic, 15 of balsam of tolu, to be dissolved in 25 of absolute alcohol, and 80 of ether. Either of these solutions is suitable for the dispensing-counter. The pills are placed in a covered pot, a few drops of the varnish, sufficient to wet all the pills, are dropped upon them, and the pot rotated so as to cover all the pills equally. They are then transferred to a pill-tile or any other earthenware surface, so that they may be detached from each other ; occasionally they are turned until the coating is quite hard.

Keratine Coating.

This is of recent introduction, and is used for pills which are intended to pass the stomach undissolved, the keratine being insoluble in the gastric juice. The method originated with Dr. Unna, of Hamburg. Only oily excipients should be used, and the pills should be covered with a thin layer of cacao-butter previous to applying the keratine solution, which is made by removing from horn all that is soluble in pepsin and hydrochloric acid. The residue is dissolved in solution of ammonia, and evaporated until only a trace of ammonia is left, the gum-like liquid which remains being the coating solution, and several thin coatings of this are imparted to the pills.

Concentric Coated Pills.

These have been proposed by Dr. Mortimer Granville, and the following formula will show what they are and how prepared :—

> Barbaloin . . . . gr. xxiv.
> Ext. Cascaræ sagradæ . . . . gr. xxiv.
> Iridin . . . . gr. xii.
> Fiant pilulæ xii.

Make the aloin into a stiff mass with as little excipient as possible ; cut into pills and coat with gelatine (hard). Then roll each pill in 2 grains of extract of cascara sagrada, and coat with keratine solution (two coatings) ; finally make the iridin into a mass, divide into 12 portions, and roll each portion round a pill ; varnish or coat with gelatine. The iridin portion of the pill is supposed to dissolve in the stomach, where it is most wanted; the keratine coating dissolves only when it reaches the duodenum, and the barbaloin portion begins to dissolve in the intestines, where its action is manifested.

TABELLÆ AND PASTILS.

FROM a paper by Mr. Harold Wyatt (*The Chemist and Druggist*, February 25, 1888), we extract the following hints regarding the manufacture of tabellæ and pastils, preparations now frequently required to be made extemporaneously on the physician's order.

Tabellæ are lozenges similar in composition to the nitro-glycerine tablets of the Pharmacopœia, so far as their basis is concerned, this being composed of cacao (containing its fixed oil), sweetened with sugar, and held together by means of tragacanth powder, water or proof spirit being used as an excipient, and the mass flavoured with essence of vanilla or rose.

According to the 'Physicians' Pharmacopœia,' the method of preparing is as follows:—The cacao and other ingredients, including the medicine to be administered, are rubbed together in a mortar, massed, in the same way as a pill-mass, with the liquid excipient, and cut into pills on a pill-machine. Each pill is then taken, dusted with a powder of equal parts powdered sugar and arrowroot to prevent sticking, and placed in a tube of brass or wood standing vertically on a tile, an accurately-fitting piston of wood giving a round form to the lozenge on being forced down the tube on the top of the pill.

The tablets may also be turned out without the mould, by simply placing the mass on the cutter of the pill-machine after piping, and pressing down the upper cutter upon it, oblong or square tablets resulting, according to the amount of mass used.

For most medicines this process answers admirably, yet there are some which could be administered in lozenge form were it not for their nauseous taste, which requires an amount of cacao and sugar to disguise scarcely compatible with the dimensions of an ordinary lozenge. In such cases Mr. Wyatt recommends glycyrrhizin, the sweet principle of liquorice-root, and saccharin .as substitutes for the sugar. He finds, for example, that 5 grains of antipyrin are rendered almost tasteless by $\frac{1}{3}$ grain of glycyrrhizin, and that the intense bitterness of strophanthus is covered by the addition of $\frac{1}{6}$ grain of saccharin to every 5 minims of tincture in the tablet.

Tablets sweetened with saccharin may be used freely in diabetes and other diseases, in which the administration of ordinary sugar lozenges would be attended with injurious results.

Another improvement in the preparation of tabellæ suggested by Mr. Wyatt is the use of a warm mortar to melt the cacao, in which state the powders can be more easily incorporated. In the original paper formulæ are given for the following :—

Tabellæ Acidi Arseniosi, each containing $\frac{1}{100}$ grain of arsenious acid.

Tabellæ Aconiti, each containing $2\frac{1}{2}$ minims of tincture of aconite.

Tabellæ Antipyrin, each containing 5 grains of antipyrin.

Tabellæ Belladonnæ, each containing 5 minims of tincture of belladonna.

Tabellæ Caffeinæ, each containing 1 grain of caffeine.

Tabellæ Cerii et Bismuthi, each containing 2 grains of cerium oxalate and 2 grains of bismuth ammonio-citrate.

Tabellæ Gelsemii, each containing $2\frac{1}{2}$ minims of liquid extract of gelsemium.

Tabellæ Hamamelidis, each containing 5 minims of liquid extract of hamamelis.

Tabellæ Nitroglycerini, each containing $\frac{1}{100}$ grain of nitroglycerine.

Tabellæ Strophanthi, each containing $2\frac{1}{2}$ minims of tincture of strophanthus.

The following formula will serve as an example of how the foregoing are made :—

Tabellæ Acidi Arseniosi.

Trituration of arsenic (1 in 100) . . .	48 grains
Cacao	70 ,,
Tragacanth powder	24 ,,
Saccharin	1 ,,
Alcohol	30 minims
Essence of vanilla	24 ,,
Distilled water	30 ,,

Place the cacao in a warm mortar; when liquefied add the powders, previously well rubbed together, and, after the mass has set, powder it with the aid of the alcohol and essence of vanilla, mass with the water, and divide into forty-eight tablets.

Pastils are soft, jelly-like jujubes, variously medicated, made from a gelatine and glycerine base, called in the Throat Hospital Pharmacopœia 'Glyco-gelatine,' which is made according to the following form :—

Gelatine	1 oz.
Glycerine	2½ ,, by weight
Orange-flower water	2½ ,, ,,
Ammoniacal solution of carmine . . .	a sufficiency

Cut the gelatine into shreds and soak in the orange-flower water for two hours; then transfer to a water-bath and heat with the glycerine until the gelatine is dissolved. Colour with the carmine solution, and pour into an oiled tray to cool.

The above-mentioned Pharmacopœia gives no formula for the solution of carmine, but 30 minims of one made as follows is enough for 6 oz. of glyco-gelatine :—

Carmine	30 grains
Solution of ammonia	a sufficiency

Dissolve the carmine in 6 drachms of the ammonia, filter, and wash the filter with more ammonia until 1 fluid oz. has been collected.

The medication of the pastils is accomplished by melting an ounce of glyco-gelatine on a water-bath, adding the medicine, previously rubbed to a thick syrup with glycerine, if a powder, stirring until nearly cool, and pouring into an oiled mould; cutting the mass into 24 pastils when cold. A suitable mould for small quantities is one with sides soldered on, square in shape, 3 inches by 3 inches, divided into 36 squares by means of deeply impressed lines on the under side, these causing the finished pastils to have a slightly rounded surface, the lines leaving a series of deep grooves, which serve as a guide to cutting.

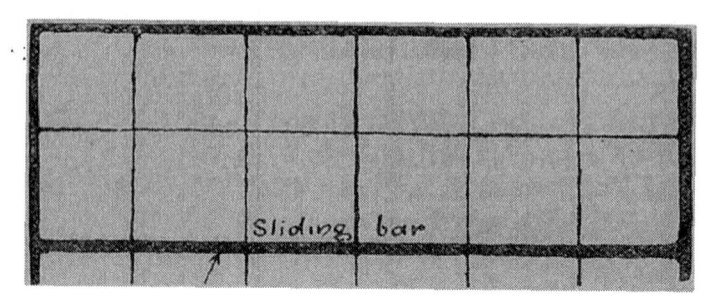

An excellent mould is also made from a square piece of plate-glass with narrow slips of plate-glass cemented on its three sides as shown in the figure. The square is divided into smaller squares by means of grooved lines, and a piece of glass is provided to slip up to any row required, there to be secured by means of a piece of cork, thus serving to give the requisite surface. The diagram shows part of the plate arranged for a dozen pastils. The plate having previously been slightly oiled, the pastil mass is poured into it, and when it sets the glyco-gelatine sheet is removed, when it is found that on the under surface are ridges corresponding to the grooves in the plate. All that remains to be done is to cut through these ridges with a pair of scissors, and the pastils are finished.

Flavours for the pastils other than orange-flower water are the fruit-juices, tolu, and glycyrrhizin. Rose or cinnamon water may be used instead of orange-flower water, and in the same proportion, whilst 2 fluid drachms of cherry-laurel water with $2\frac{1}{4}$ oz. of distilled water impart a pleasant almond flavour. Raspberry juice may be used in the same proportion as orange-flower water, lime-juice in the proportion of half juice and half distilled water. Tolu $1\frac{1}{4}$ part with 30 of glycerine and 6 of water heated over a water-bath for an hour, filtered on cooling, and made up to 36 fluid parts by the addition of glycerine : this also is a nice flavour. Glycyrrhizin, 24 grains, dissolved in the water used to soak the gelatine, imparts an excellent liquorice flavour, very useful to hide the taste of ammonium chloride.

CAPSULES.

A GROWING disposition on the part of medical men to prescribe nauseous medicines in capsules makes it necessary for
the dispenser to be acquainted with the details of the operation
of capsule-making. The requisites are moulds, or olives, as
the French call them. These are egg or olive shaped, solid
heads of iron or britannia metal, each of which is fixed upon
a metal rod; a dozen or more of the moulds are fixed into a
slab of wood or cork, with perforations for the purpose, and at
the back of the slab, in the centre, a handle is fixed. A good
slab or holder may be
made from a large cork
bung. The appearance
of the moulds fixed on
the holder is seen in the
accompanying figure.
The moulds are the only
part of the requisite
apparatus which are not
home-made. A slab of
wood with quarter-inch

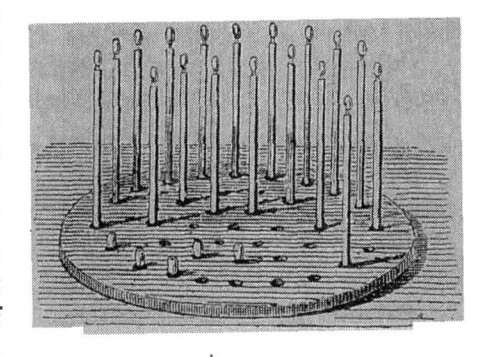

perforations bored with a centre-bit (the holder as shown for
example), or even a suppository mould, serves to support the
capsules in the process of filling, and most liquids are poured
into the capsules by means of an ordinary glass syringe.
The 15-minim capsule is the common size, but the size
may vary from 5 minims to 1 or even 2 drachms. If the
moulds are made locally the chemist should supply the
moulder with the shape from which to work. For this pur-

pose use clean yellow wax, 15 grains for each 15-minim mould; warm the wax and form it into the proper shape, with as smooth a surface as possible. The moulder will of course make the metal mould perfectly smooth; the slightly greater bulk, proportionately, of the wax allows a fair margin for this purpose.

Capsules are either hard or soft. The former were the first introduced, but the latter are now deservedly the more popular, for they are more easily swallowed. The solution for hard capsules is made according to the following formula, although the quantity of liquid used in this and other cases must vary with the quality of the gelatine :—

	Oz.
Gelatine	6
Gum acacia	1
Powdered sugar	1
Water	5

Steep the gelatine in the water, when soft add the gum and sugar, and heat until dissolved, removing any scum which rises to the surface.

Various forms have been proposed for the soft capsules. The following have been found to give good flexible masses :—

	Parts
(1) Gelatine, gum acacia, sugar	each 30
Honey	10
Water	100

Make a solution as above.

	Parts
(2) Gelatine	25
Glycerine	10
Sugar	8
Water	45

Steep the gelatine in the water, add the sugar and glycerine, and dissolve by the heat of a water-bath.

A stock of No. 2 may be kept and dissolved as required by means of a water-bath. To make the capsules, have the gelatine mixture melted and heated to 104° F.; prepare the moulds by oiling them very slightly with olive oil. This is best done by oiling a soft cloth, such as a piece of lint, and applying this over the whole of the mould surface and a little way up the supporting-rod. Lift the mould-holder by the handle and immerse the moulds completely in the gelatine mixture ; in a few seconds remove steadily and begin to rotate the moulds in a circular fashion, so that the gelatine may set perfectly even. A little practice suffices to make the operator perfect in this operation. In a couple of minutes the gelatine has set sufficiently to allow the whole to be set aside. In about a quarter of an hour the capsules may be removed by grasping each lightly with the finger and thumb and gently pulling off. Place each one upon its closed end in one or other of the supporters already described, and when the whole have been removed cut off their tails with a pair of scissors. They are now ready for filling, and in the case of liquids this is simply done with a syringe; for powders use a small funnel made of paper. The open end is closed by dipping a glass rod in the liquefied gelatine solution and placing the drop which it removes upon the open end. Sometimes a superior finish is given to the capsules by afterwards dipping this end of the capsule halfway up in the gelatine solution and drying rapidly, but one must be an adept before this refinement is attempted. After they are finished it is necessary to expose the capsules to the air for a few hours, in order to dry them thoroughly.

POWDERS.

THE method which is almost universally followed is to mix the powders in a glass mortar, very cautious dispensers also sifting. Indiscriminate use of mortar and pestle is bad. Here, for example, is a prescription of Sir Morell Mackenzie's, which was in the first instance dispensed by a well-known West-end pharmacist, and gave satisfaction :—

Bismuthi subnit.	gr. $\frac{1}{8}$
Pulv. catechu	gr. $\frac{1}{12}$
Morphinæ hydrochlor.	gr. $\frac{1}{16}$

The powders were used for insufflation in a case of chronic sore-throat. The second pharmacist who dispensed the prescription is an ardent advocate of the mortar-and-pestle method, and he lost a customer by the practice of his principle. The third with his spatula mixed the powders on a powder-paper, and the patient no longer sent to London in order to get the prescription dispensed. The complaint made of the powders sent out by the second pharmacist was that they had a lumpy feeling in the throat, and did not adhere so kindly as those supplied by the first and third dispensers. No doubt the heat of friction had caused aggregation of the catechu with the other ingredients.

It has been shown by Mr. Boa of Edinburgh that the method of mixing materially affects the miscibility of powders. The general conclusion arrived at from Mr. Boa's experiments is that powders mixed on paper and sifted are more readily miscible in water than those which have been rubbed up in a mortar and sifted. For example, we may quote two instances in which this effect may be readily observed :—

Pulv. rhei	gr. x
Pulv. cinnamom.	gr. vj.
Magnes. levis	gr. xx.

If this powder be rubbed up in a mortar it diffuses in water with exceeding difficulty, whereas when mixed on paper it diffuses quickly.

Pepsin	gr. ij.
Bismuth. alb.	gr. v.
Magnes. carb.	gr. iij.
Pulv. aromat.	gr. j.

When these are rubbed up in a mortar, and sifted, they can be mixed in water only with considerable difficulty, but when mixed on paper the same difficulty is not experienced.

The following powder is a distinct exception to the foregoing :—

Sulphur. præcip.	gr. xv.
Guaiac. resin.	gr. x.
Magnesiæ	gr. xx.

The most readily miscible powder is here obtained by rubbing the guaiacum and magnesia well together before adding the sulphur. If the powders are mixed on paper they will scarcely mix with water.

It is quite evident that there is an art in powder-making, as there is in pill-making, the only difference being that in the former case dissatisfaction is experienced by the customer, in the latter by the dispenser—a sufficient reason, therefore, to call forth the care and ingenuity of the dispenser in mixing powders.

In the great majority of cases, where limited quantities are ordered, say under 2 drachms—such, for example, as one or two dozen of powders—no better or quicker method of mixing the powders can be adopted than the spatula and a sheet of white paper. The ingredients ordered in smallest quantity should be first thoroughly incorporated, and the larger quantities added gradually.

Salts which are likely to mutually decompose each other must be mixed in a perfectly dry condition, and must be stirred together lightly in the mortar. Instances are tartrate of potash with sulphate of soda, tartrate of potash with muriate of ammonia, nitrate of potash with salicylate of soda. Effervescing lemonade-powder should be mixed by first rubbing together the tartaric acid with the sugar in a previously warmed mortar and then stirring in the bicarbonate of soda very lightly. The powders should not be dried at a temperature above 30° C., or they are more liable to absorb moisture afterwards.

Hygroscopic Substances, such as acetate, carbonate, and citrate of potash and iodide of sodium, ought not to be prescribed as powders, but if prescribed in bulk they keep fairly well. If prescribed in powders, each dose should be folded up in waxed paper, that again being covered with ordinary powder-paper. Do not attempt the reverse way.

Preservation of Hygroscopic Drugs.—When the drying of any drug has been efficiently accomplished, it should at once be stored in a proper receptacle, not left, as is often the case, to reabsorb moisture and collect dust. Shop-drawers, so generally used for storage, are in the main of but little value, their contents often becoming mouldy and covered with dust, besides being easy of access to insects and other pests. Wide-mouthed bottles and stone jars are good vessels for storage ; they should have accurately fitting stoppers or corks ; the corks may be advantageously soaked in melted paraffin to render them air-tight. Powders of squills and ammoniacum can be kept from aggregating by suspending in the bottle a bag of quicklime fastened to the cork or stopper. The lime absorbs any moisture that may enter.

No Guess-work.—In dividing powders *weigh each one ;* division by guess-work is considered sufficient for the rejection of a candidate at the minor examination.

General Directions.—When the physician orders salts like iodide of potassium, or roots like gentian, with directions for their solution or infusion by the patient himself, the dispenser should destroy their identity by the pestle before sending them out.

Powders containing ammonium carbonate should be wrapped in waxed paper, and be put into a bottle as well.

Powders for lotions, injections, etc., should be sent out in a different coloured paper from that used in other cases. A coloured paper is useful as distinguishing at once between an internal and external remedy.

Administering Powders.—It is the practice of many parents to give powders to children mixed with jam; there is no objection to this, provided the ingredients are compatible with the jam; but it should be borne in mind that many children's powders contain magnesia or carbonate of soda, and the acid present in all jams would combine with and alter the action of a portion of these ingredients. The simplest way to give a powder is to make a small draught of it with sugar and water. Treacle is sometimes recommended, but is objectionable in some cases owing to its alkalinity.

SUPPOSITORIES, BOUGIES, AND PESSARIES.

THE use of these is well known and requires no explanation. The bases in common use for forming them are generally of three kinds : (1) Fatty, such as cacao-butter, which is the favourite ; (2) saponaceous, as in the official soap suppositories ; and (3) gelatine—in this class may be included dextrin and similar substances. The basis should be sufficiently hard not to melt in the fingers when handled, and yet become perfectly soft or liquid when introduced into the body. Bougies are cylindrical pipes varying in diameter from $\frac{1}{12}$th to $\frac{1}{6}$th of an inch, and are from $2\frac{1}{2}$ to $6\frac{1}{2}$ inches in length—a bougie $2\frac{1}{2}$ inches long and $\frac{1}{8}$th inch in diameter weighs about 15 grains. Suppositories seldom exceed 15 grains in weight—that is, they fill the same space as 15 grains of water, and are 1 inch long and $\frac{1}{4}$ inch in diameter. The common shape is shown in fig. 1, p. 109. Pessaries are merely very large suppositories weighing 2 drachms or thereabouts. Electro-plated gun-metal moulds of the sizes indicated are used for moulding the three forms mentioned, but bougies are also moulded or piped with a machine resembling a pill-piping machine. Clay moulds are made by pressing oiled pieces of wood the shape of the suppository in plastic clay and withdrawing them ; but this makes a very clumsy method. A similar plan is to form moulds with tinfoil upon a shaped piece of wood, and place the hollow cones in a box of French chalk or other powder.

For **Bougie-Moulds** an elastic-gum bougie is generally taken as a model on which to wrap the tinfoil ; but the bougie being of the same thickness nearly all its length, there is considerable difficulty in drawing off the mould from the model, the sides of the mould being drawn together. This trouble may be obviated by using a piece of glass tubing same size as a No. 8 bougie. First draw out the end to a point and cut it off about an eighth of an inch from where the narrowing begins, then fuse again until the end is rounded off as the bougie is to be, taking care not to allow the aperture to close. This tube now forms the model upon which to shape the tinfoil moulds. The tinfoil slips more easily from the glass than from elastic

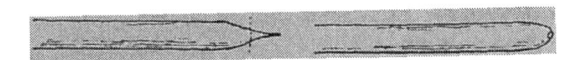

gum, and the little hole at the apex allows air to enter as the tube is withdrawn. This plan serves well for unusual sizes.

Moulding with the fingers is also done, and in many cases must be resorted to. Finely powdered starch should in this case be used to prevent sticking to the fingers. The Pharmacopœia now directs cacao-butter only, instead of the mixture of cacao-butter, lard, and wax, to be used for suppositories. This is a great improvement, but for dispensing purposes, especially in the summer months, it is still necessary to add a little white wax—say about 1 grain to 10 grains of cacao-butter. Whatever the basis may be, it is important that it should not be heated too high; do not by any means heat the dish containing the basis over a strong flame. It is preferable to do all the liquefying operations by means of a water-bath.

We give here an illustration of a small handy water-bath, which is exceedingly useful n making suppositories, small quantities of ointments, or for use in any 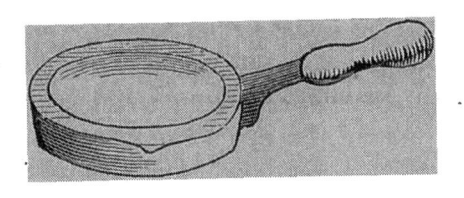 operation which requires moderate heat to be raised quickly.

The bath may be made of tin or copper. The diameter at the outside may be 4 inches, with a ½-inch rim returning towards the inside and provided with a small outlet for pouring out the water. The depth should be about 1 inch. The handle is best made of wood, so that the bath may be lifted without fear of burning the hand. Half an ounce of

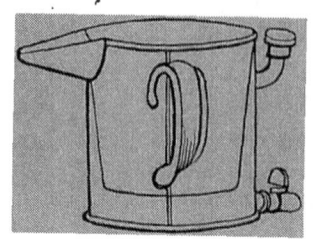 water is sufficient to use for a small operation. A series of rings may be got so as to take small dishes, such as watch-glasses. A bath of the size described, made of copper, costs about half a crown. Another excellent bath is that designed by Mr. Learoyd, the construction of which is shown in this drawing. The feature of this is the long lip, which permits the suppository-mass to be poured into the mould without loss.

THE MANUFACTURE OF SUPPOSITORIES.

Theobroma Suppositories.—It is customary to make prescription suppositories with cacao-butter unless there is an order to the contrary. The following is the plan to adopt : Having weighed out the amount of fat required, shave it into shreds and melt as previously directed. As soon as this is done place the powdered ingredients—extracts should previously be rubbed smooth with a few drops of water, or, better, with a little powdered curd soap—on a slab, and add only just sufficient of the melted fat to make the ingredients into a smooth paste, then add more, taking great care that it is not too hot. When about half has been added stop, return to the dish the mixture of fat and medicament, and stir constantly till nearly cold ; if lumpy, hold the dish above the water-bath, and rub the lumps down. It is very important not to reliquefy the mass. When the lumps are thoroughly removed, pour into the mould ; perhaps only four or six holes are filled before the mass is too solid to pour out. This matters little, as, in order to soften, it is only necessary to hold the dish again above the water-bath, stirring till it seems sufficiently fluid to pour about six more, and so on.

Mr. Martindale has spoken highly of a mixture of equal parts of stearic and oleic acids as a substitute for cacao-butter ; the advantages which he claims for it are that—(1) the mixture has a very low fusing-point, and readily melts at the temperature of the body ; (2) the suppositories leave the mould without difficulty ; (3) it has the advantage, besides being a solvent of such alkaloids as pure morphine, atropine, cocaine, etc., of being, at least as far as the oleic acid is concerned, readily absorbed by the skin and mucous membrane; (4) on account of the partial crystallisation of some of the stearic acid, the suppositories are firm, and can be placed in their position without difficulty, not being elastic, brittle, or yielding in any way ; and (5) the proportions of stearic and oleic acids can be varied to suit the temperature of summer or winter, and also the other ingredients prescribed with them. These opinions were expressed many years ago, but cacao-butter has maintained its pre-eminence.

Pouring the Mass into the Mould.—Complaints are frequently made of the difficulty of getting nicely finished suppositories and pessaries from gun-metal moulds. The supposition may be wrong, but from experience we are inclined to impute much of the difficulty to an imperfect knowledge of the conditions regulating the expansion and contraction of both mould and substance used in their production. If, for example, the substance (say, oil of theobroma) be poured into the moulds at a temperature much above 140° or below 130°, the melting-point being 124°, it will be found that the suppositories, if they come out at all, will in either case be broken and imperfect, for this reason—that above the melting-point the oil of theobroma does not expand under different increments of heat in the same degree with the metal. Consequently, the higher the temperature of the theobroma the more is the metal expanded, which, cooling first, contracts on the ball like a vice. This, together probably with unequal cooling, produces unequal elasticities within the suppository, which sufficiently accounts for the moulds refusing to give up their contents, as well as for the cracked and uneven appearance of the suppositories. On the other hand, should the theobroma be poured into the mould at too low a temperature, the metal at once cools it to such an extent that contraction within the mass cannot take place, and the same result ensues as in the previous case, but from the very opposite cause. The proper plan, therefore, is to heat the substance to the temperature already indicated, to smear the moulds with one or other of the liquids which are mentioned below, and pour the melted substance quickly in. If expeditiously and properly done, the suppositories, when cool, should slip from the mould without the least trouble, having a beautiful polished finish, and, what is more important

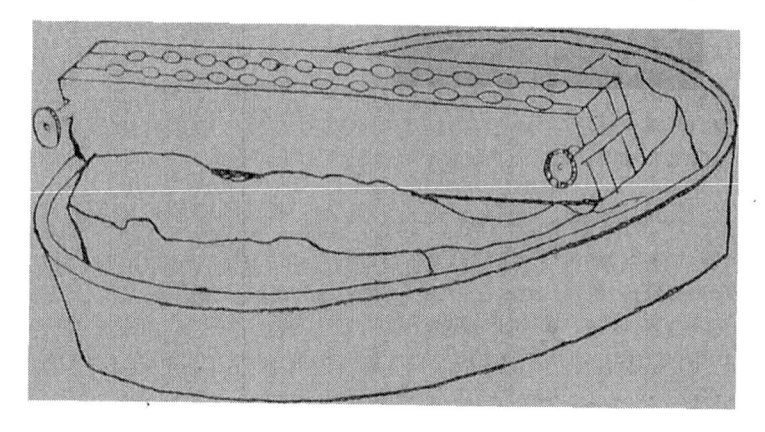

still, having a uniform composition and structure, and not with the active medicinal agent all concentrated at the apex, as is always the case when the heat applied has been excessive.

The mould should be quite clean, chilled with ice or cold water; just before filling it should be wiped with a piece of sponge or lint moistened with soap-liniment; very little should be used, but every part inside the mould must be coated. A fluid mixture of soft soap, glycerine, and water is sometimes used instead of soap-liniment, and some dispensers prefer to use olive-oil, but on the whole soap-liniment is the best.

The figure shows how the suppository-mould is generally cooled by placing on ice after it has been cleaned and sponged with soap-liniment. The melted base may be poured in while the mould is in this position.

The Gelatine Basis is a very valuable one, and is serviceable where a fatty basis is objectionable. *Suppositories* of this basis can be made much more easily and quickly than theobroma suppositories. The mould should be cold, clean, and quite dry ; then thinly coated inside with almond oil. When turned out the suppositories should be wiped with a dry cloth in order to remove the oil, or placed for this purpose on a sheet of filtering-paper. A mortar or slab is not convenient to use with this basis ; it is simply melted in a dish, and the medicament stirred in until thoroughly dissolved or diffused. The gelatine basis is well adapted for the exhibition of alkaloids and aqueous extracts, but not for tannin, carbolic acid, or bromide and iodide of potassium.

The ' Extra Pharmacopœia ' gives the following formula for the basis :—

> Gelatine . . . . 1 oz.
>
> Immerse in 4 oz. of water for a few seconds, drain, and in half an hour add—
>
> Glycerine (by weight) . . . . . 4 oz.
>
> Dissolve on a water-bath. Should weigh 6 oz.

Another satisfactory formula is :—

> Gelatine . . . . ℥j.
> Glycerine . . . . ℥ij.
> Distilled water . . . . ℥ij.

Wash the gelatine in cold water, macerate in the distilled water until soft, add the glycerine, and dissolve in a water-bath.

It should be observed, however, that one mass is not universally applicable, because various medicaments act upon it in diverse ways, rendering the suppositories too hard or too soft, as the case may be. Herr G. H. Ochse, who has had considerable experience with this basis, has formulated his views, and from his communication (*Pharm Rundsch.*) we abstract the following hints :—

Where gelatine preparations are frequently dispensed it is best to have a definite mass in stock. This is made in large quantities or small, according to the requirements of the pharmacist. After removing the scum from the solution the latter is poured into bottles, and when thoroughly cooled covered with alcohol to prevent it from becoming mouldy. When wanted for use the bottle is placed in a water-bath and the required quantity poured off. The mass is made as follows : The accurately weighed gelatine is allowed to macerate over night in distilled water, and strained through a sieve. The gelatine adhering to the sieve is collected, the whole placed in a tared porcelain dish, and sufficient water added to make the weight four or five times as much as the original quantity of gelatine used. The dish is placed on the upper ring of a retort-stand and heated over wire gauze with a gas or spirit-lamp flame, care being taken not to burn the gelatine. The glycerine is added and the whole evaporated to the consistency required, viz.—

I. Gelatine 20 parts, water 80 parts, glycerine 40 parts ; evaporated to 60 parts. Intended for preparations kept in stock and for those which are to retain their transparency.

II. Gelatine 10 parts, water 40 parts, glycerine 15 parts ; evaporated to 25 parts. For hygroscopic drugs, for bougies of perchloride of iron (made by dissolving 1 part of ferric chloride in 9 parts of water, and adding to 19 parts of the mass), for tannin suppositories (0·2 per cent.—but this recommendation is opposed to theory), and for vaginal pessaries containing iodide or bromide of potassium, bromide, chloride, or salicylate of sodium, and ergotin. Chloral hydrate suppositories are made with this mass, the hydrate being dissolved in as little water as possible.

III. Gelatine 10 parts, water 40 parts, glycerine 20 parts ; evaporated to 50 parts. For suppositories generally, also in special cases, as for carbolic acid (and similar medicaments soluble in a small quantity of alcohol), which are made by adding 3 parts of carbolic acid, previously dissolved in alcohol, to 7 parts of glycerine and 50 parts of this mass. To make alum bougies, liquefy 25 parts of the mass and 10 parts of distilled water on a water-bath. To this add a *hot* solution of 7 parts alum, 10 parts glycerine, and 5 parts distilled water. The whole is then evaporated with slight agitation to 35 parts. The mixture becomes thick and turbid on adding the solution of alum, but, on heating over a water-bath and stirring carefully, it soon becomes clear and transparent. Hot water must be added from time to time to replace that lost by evaporation.

IV. Gelatine 10 parts, water 40 parts, glycerine 30 parts ; evaporated to 60 parts. This mass is used for certain vaginal pessaries, and for urethral bougies, especially those containing sulphate of zinc, sulphate of copper, nitrate of silver, extract of opium, hydrochlorate of morphine, bichloride of mercury. One part of any of them is first dissolved in a little water, and then added to 99 parts of mass and poured into moulds. If it is desired to make a large quantity of sulphate of copper bougies, it is best to mix not more than the mould will hold at a time, because by frequently heating the mass the bougies acquire a yellowish-green instead of a blue-green colour.

V. Gelatine 30 parts, water 120 parts, glycerine 15 parts ; evaporated to 104 parts. Used for bougies containing a large percentage of powdered drugs insoluble in water or alcohol. Thus 50 per cent. bougies of iodoform are made by adding 27 parts of powdered iodoform to 54 parts of mass. When taken from the mould the bougies are placed in a drying closet until they weigh about two-thirds of their original weight.

These hints also serve for the extemporaneous preparation of any kind of gelatine suppositories, bougies, etc

HINTS FOR SPECIAL CASES.

Chloral Hydrate must not be heated with the cacao-butter, otherwise the mass will not harden. To make the suppository beat together 5 grains of chloral hydrate and 10 grains of cacao-butter, and press into the mould.

Cocaine.—The hydrochlorate, but preferably the pure alkaloid, can be dissolved in oleic acid and added to the prepared base. It is preferable in the case of all alkaloids to combine them in suppositories as oleates, made extemporaneously. Of course when the gelatine base is used this does not apply.

Green Extracts and Tannin.—The slightest degree of over-heating coagulates the tannin into hard lumps. The same remark applies to powdered galls.

We have never had any difficulty with even large quantities of green extracts by taking care to soften the extracts with water, and to mix them intimately with the melted, but not too hot, fat, as in the following case :—

Ext. belladonnæ	.	.	.	.	.	. gr. v.
Potassii bromid.	.	.	.	.	.	. gr. x.
Ol. theobrom.	.	.	.	.	.	. q.s.

Fiat suppos. Mitte vj.

Powder the bromide as finely as possible, and place it on a tile; rub down the extract on the tile with 3 to 5 drops of water. Melt 50 grains of cacao-butter and 5 grains of white wax over a water-bath, and rub up more than one-half of it with the medicaments on the tile. Then transfer to the dish containing the rest of the basis, mix expertly, slightly heating if necessary, and pour into the mould.

The following prescription would be a simple one to compound were it not for the presence of the tannin, so that it is inadvisable to melt the basis :—

Ext. bellad.	.	.	.	.	.	. gr. iij.
Plumb. acet.	.	.	.	.	.	. gr. ij.
Ac. tannic.	.	.	.	.	.	. gr. iv.
Ol. theobrom. q.s. ut ft. suppos. gr. xv.						

Mitte vj.

The simplest method of dispensing these is to take 54 grains of cacao-butter for the six suppositories and shave it into shreds; soften the extract in a warm mortar with a few drops of water, mix the butter intimately with this, add the tannin and the lead acetate, each in fine powder, and work up like a pill-mass; weigh out each suppository and press into the mould.

The annexed figure shows a section of a mould which is very useful for making such suppositories as those in the last-mentioned prescription. The mould proper is formed, it will be seen, of two hollowed-out pieces of metal or hard wood, wedge-shaped externally, so as to fit into the stout ring. The weighed quantity of material is pressed well into the mould by means of the stopper, as shown.

We quote the following on account of the large dose of extract of opium, rather than for any unusual inherent difficulty which it presents :—

Ext. opii	.	.	.	.	.	.	3 grains.
,, belladonnæ	.	.	.	.	.	I	,,
Ol. theobromæ	.	.	.	.	.	20	,,

Fiat suppos.

It is advisable in this case to use 18 grains of ol. theobromæ and 2 grains of white wax (the addition of wax in all these cases is beneficial). Rub down the extracts in a mortar with sufficient water to make a smooth soft paste; add half of the fatty matter to this gradually, so that a perfect mixture may be obtained. Then transfer it to the dish, and dissolve in the remainder of the fat, aiding the process by the heat of a water-bath if necessary.

Hamamelis Suppositories.—These may be made with the liquid extract of the British Pharmaceutical Conference Formulary—5 minims in each suppository, with a cacao-butter basis, as well as with hamamelin. The liquid extract should be evaporated to one half its bulk.

Salts in Suppositories.—The settling of the active ingredient of some suppositories at the apex has already been referred to. We have seen bromide of potassium suppositories sent out with all the bromide at the extreme point, forming a hard, gritty, almost insoluble mass, which must have been not only exceedingly disagreeable to the patient, but even dangerous. This is perfectly inexcusable, and need never occur if care be taken to have the substance first thoroughly impalpable, and then incorporated with a part of the theobroma, previous to adding to the melted portion at a temperature a little over the melting-point. There is, moreover, another evil attending the overheating of the mixture, where powders of a ponderous nature, such as bromide and iodide of potassium, or acetate and iodide of lead, are ordered, namely, the impossibility of an equal division of the substance where a number of suppositories are being simultaneously made. The powder falls to the bottom of the dish, owing to the fluidity of the theobroma, and no amount of stirring or dexterity of manipulation will ensure its equal distribution.

It is in this class of suppositories that the gelatine basis has the advantage—for instance, in the case of iodine, which should have a little potassium iodide added to render it soluble.

Iodi	gr. ij.
Potas. iodidi	gr. iss.
Gelat. et glycer.	ℨiss.

Finely powder the iodine and iodide, stir with a *little* of the melted basis until entirely dissolved, then add the rest of the basis.

Ergotin Suppositories are very frequently prescribed, and present little difficulty when the dose is 3 grains or under, but 5-grain suppositories are not uncommon, and we have seen as much as 8 grains prescribed. An excellent suppository is made with the No. 2 gelatine basis, the ergotin being thinned, if necessary, with a little water and added to the melted basis. With cacao-butter the procedure is the same as with green extracts, a little wax being added to the cacao-butter, and care being taken to incorporate the ergotin with half of the melted fat.

Hollow suppositories have for some years been introduced among the American physicians. They are made in the sizes and forms shown in the engraving, with stoppers, and are formed of cacao-butter. They only require the medicament to be inserted. The convenience of these cases is obvious. Size o is for children, and can also be used for the ear or nose.

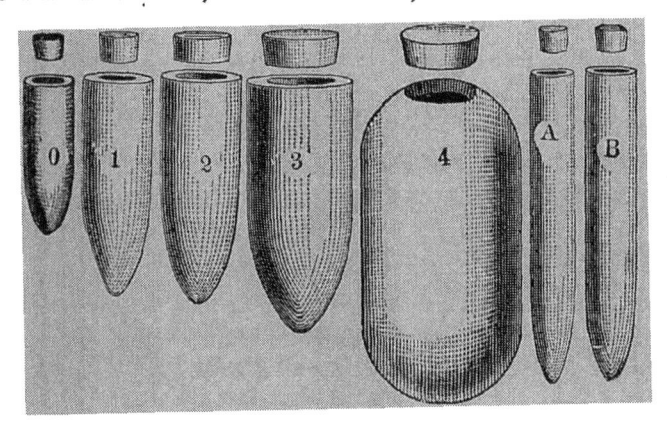

Nos. 1, 2, and 3 are for the rectum. Nos. 3 and 4 can be used for the introduction of nourishment per rectum. Nos. 4 and 5 (the latter not shown in this drawing—a circular suppository) are for vaginal application. A and B are for application to parts of the urethra, the uterus, or the nostrils. They were brought into commerce by Messrs. Hall & Ruckel, of New York. Messrs. S. Maw, Son & Thompson supply them in England.

STRENGTHS OF BOUGIES, PESSARIES, AND SUPPOSITORIES.

Bougies.—The following are given by Mr. Martindale as the strengths generally used for those with a cacao-butter basis:

Belladonna (root extract)	. . . .	gr. $\frac{1}{4}$
Bismuth oxychloride	. . . .	gr. x.
Cocaine	. . . . . .	gr. $\frac{1}{2}$
Eucalyptus oil	. . . . .	♏x.
Iodoform	. . . . . .	gr. v.
,,	(also with eucalyptus oil, ♏x).	

Lead acetate	gr. $\frac{1}{2}$-gr. j.
Tannic acid	gr. j.
Zinc chloride.	gr. $\frac{1}{4}$-gr. $\frac{1}{2}$
Zinc sulphate	gr. $\frac{1}{2}$-gr. j.

Nasal Bougies of Glycerine :—

Acidi carbolici	gr. $\frac{1}{2}$
Cocainæ hydrochloratis	gr. $\frac{1}{6}$
Cupri sulphatis	gr. $\frac{1}{10}$-gr. $\frac{1}{6}$
Iodoformi	gr. $\frac{1}{2}$
Zinci sulphatis	gr. $\frac{1}{10}$

Pessaries and Suppositories.—The following are the strengths as ordered by leading physicians :—

	Pessaries	Suppositories
Acetate of lead. . . .	7$\frac{1}{2}$ grs.	—
,, ,, and opium .	5 grs. and 2 grs.	3 grs. and 1 gr.
Aloin	— . . .	. 1 gr.
Alum	10 grs. . .	—
Alum and catechu . .	10 grs. of each .	—
Atropine	$\frac{1}{20}$ gr. . .	. $\frac{1}{20}$ gr.
Belladonna extract . .	5 grs. . .	$\frac{1}{2}$ gr. to 2 grs.
Bismuth subnitrate . .	15 grs. . .	. 10 grs.
Boric acid . . .	10 grs. . .	. 3 grs.
Bromide of potassium .	10 grs. . .	—
Carbolic acid . . .	2 grs. . .	. 1 gr.
Chloral	— . .	. 5 grs.
Cocaine	$\frac{1}{2}$ gr. . .	, $\frac{1}{2}$ gr.
Gallic acid . . .	10 grs. . .	—
Gall and opium . . .	— . .	5 grs. and 1 gr.
Hamamelin . . .	— . .	. 1 gr.
Iodide of lead . . .	5 grs. . .	—
Iodide of potassium . .	10 grs. . .	—
Iodoform. . . .	5 grs. . .	—
Opium	2 grs. . .	. 1 gr.
Santonin	— . .	. 3-6 grs.
Sulphate of zinc . .	10 grs. . .	. 2 grs.
Sulphocarbolate of zinc .	10 grs. . .	—
Tannic acid . . .	10 grs. . .	. 3 grs.
Zinc oxide . . .	15 grs. . .	. 10 grs.

OINTMENTS.

GENERAL INSTRUCTIONS.

OINTMENTS are often troublesome, and therefore we may usefully summarise the principles which should guide the dispenser in making them. Powders should be added in such a state that the resulting ointment will be free from grittiness; extracts, balsams, or any fluid or semi-fluid should be added in such a state as is best fitted to produce a perfectly homogeneous mixture. In the case of powders the mortar will, in the majority of cases, be sufficient to reduce them to a fine enough state of division, but in some cases, and often with extracts, balsams, etc., a preliminary treatment with some medium, such as oil, water, or spirit, is necessary. Whatever medium is chosen it should not in any way interfere with or affect the medicinal properties of the ointment. Opium or watery extracts should be rubbed down smooth with a little water before being combined with an ointment; spirituous extracts with a little diluted spirit. Soluble salts, such as perchloride of mercury, sulphate of zinc, nitrate of silver, etc., which are likely to crystallise, are best rubbed smooth with a little oil. But very soluble or deliquescent salts, such as carbonate of potash, iodide of potassium, chloride of zinc, etc., are best rubbed down with a little water. Tartarated antimony should be mixed dry with the ointment basis.

Incorporating Liquids.—In the preparation of certain ointments where a liquid has to be added to a fatty base, and a *quasi*-emulsion has to be made, circular stirring towards the dispenser is important. The action must always be slow, and larger quantities of a liquid can be incorporated thus than the inexperienced would deem possible. A striking instance is shown in incorporating liquor plumbi subacetatis with lard. Not less remarkable is the effect on colour ; otherwise dark ointments can be rendered nearly white, and with very faint indication of the original colouring ingredient. This is the case with various shades of brown, yellow, or greenish vegetable colours, the exception being with regard to the pronounced decoloration of certain chemical salts, such as in red oxide of mercury.

Glycerine is most easily incorporated into ointments by using a mortar which has been first thoroughly warmed by hot water.

Tinctures and other spirituous substances are not easily combined with fat. Ordinary soft lard will take up one-fifth, hard lard will take up one-sixth, of its weight of tincture. To mix them, the lard or other fatty substance should be spread evenly on the bottom and sides of the mortar, and the tincture added gradually. A little soap-powder, if permissible, greatly facilitates the combination.

The following is an ointment which is rather difficult to prepare :—

> Lin. camphoræ co. . . . . . ʒij.
> Ung. potass. iod. . . . . . ʒij.
> M. Fiat unguentum.

The best method, without alteration of the formula, is to place the ointment in a mortar, add the liniment drop by drop, and stir constantly. The ammonia in the liniment combines with the fat of the ointment to form a soap, thus greatly assisting the compounding. This method requires considerable care in order to produce a creamy preparation which does not separate, and, if you fail, begin afresh, using a little soap to assist combination. Hager states that if too large a proportion of tincture be prescribed in an ointment, it may, if its active ingredients be not volatile, be treated as follows : About half of the tincture is evaporated by gentle heat in the mortar to a pasty consistence, and this is dissolved in the rest of the tincture, and then combined with the ointment. This course may be followed with tincture of opium.

There are some solids which require special treatment ; for example—

Camphor.—If time permit, the best plan in the case of the following prescription—

Camphoræ .	. . . .	℥j.
Zinci oxidi .	. . . . . .	℥ij.
Vaselini	. . . .	℥iss.

—is to powder the camphor and add it to the melted vaseline contained in a covered pot. Stir occasionally until the camphor is dissolved, then strain, and finish off the ointment in the usual way.

Chloral.—To look at, the following prescription would seem to provide for a very hard ointment :—

Chloral	. . . .	1 part
Menthol	. . . .	1 ,,
Cacao-butter	. . . . . .	4 parts
Spermaceti .	. . . . . .	2 ,,

Melt the cacao-butter and spermaceti, and when getting creamy add the chloral and menthol, previously powdered, and stir until cold. The chloral prevents the basis from becoming quite solid.

Chrysarobin ('Chrysophanic acid').—This should be dispensed dissolved, if possible, in the fatty basis of the ointment, but if there is not sufficient fat to form a perfect solution, it is preferable to rub the chrysarobin to fine powder, and gradually incorporate the solid basis with it. In making the official ointment it will be noticed that the chrysarobin dissolves perfectly in the melted basis, but on cooling a part of it crystallises out, and these crystals cause some irritation when applied to the skin. Chrysarobin is more soluble in castor-oil than in lard, and, taking advantage of this fact, Mr. J. R. Hill has proposed the following formula :—

I

Chrysarobin	.	.	.	.	.	. 20 grains .
White wax.	.	.	.	.	.	. 60 ,, .
Castor-oil .	.	.	.	.	.	. 180 ,,
Prepared lard	.	.	.	.	.	. 240 ,,
Tincture of benzoin (1 in 5)		.	.	.	. .	20 minims

Melt the wax in the castor-oil by the aid of heat, add the tincture of benzoin and the chrysarobin, and continue the heat until the latter is dissolved. Place the lard in a mortar, pour in the other ingredients while hot, mix thoroughly and continue the rubbing until cold.

Cocaine and other alkaloids are, for therapeutic reasons, best combined in ointments as oleates. For this purpose dissolve the pure alkaloid in a sufficiency of oleic acid and mix with the basis.

Extracts.—Mention has already been made of the green extracts, which should always be thinned with water and the fatty matter added to it by portions. This is the plan which should be followed in the case of the following formula :—

Unguentum Hyoscyami (Middlesex Hospital).

Ext. hyoscyami.	.	.	.	.	.	. ℥ss.
Adipis	.	.	.	.	.	. ℥ss.
Glycerini .	.	.	.	.	.	. ʒj.

In making ung. belladonnæ, B.P., from the root extract, a mixture of glycerine and water, equal parts, in the proportion of half a minim for each grain, should be used for thinning the extract.

Iodine is first rubbed down by itself, then with about its own weight of the fatty excipient. At this point a few drops of rectified spirit should be added, and the rest of the ointment then worked in. If any haloid salt, such as iodide of potassium or metallic salts, are to be combined in the ointment, the addition of spirit is superfluous, because these salts, with the addition of a little water, render the iodine easily incorporated.

Iodoform in ointments should be reduced to fine powder, and mixed with the cold basis. Heat should not be used.

Oleates, made popular in medical practice through the advocacy of Dr. John Shoemaker, of Philadelphia, are in most cases applied in ointment form, and for that reason may be considered here. It is important to remember the precaution given by Mr. H. B. Parsons, that oleates should not be melted in a metallic dish, but in porcelain basins, glass rods or bone spatulas being used to stir or mix them. If the oleates are prescribed for their local effects, and are to be diluted, vaseline is the best diluent.; on the other hand, if absorption is not to be retarded, oleic acid should by preference be used, or lard, lanoline, or fixed oil. The oleates of the alkaloids are generally employed without dilution. Most of the metallic oleates are obtainable in the powder form for use as dusting powder or for making ointments. The following are the accepted strengths of the more common oleates or oleate-ointments.

Aconitine, 1 grain ; oleic acid, 50 minims.

Aluminium.—Oleate, 1 or 2 drachms, to 1 oz. lard.

Arsenic.—Oleate, 20 grains ; lard, 1 oz.

Atropine, 1 grain ; oleic acid, 40 minims.

Bismuth Oleate is generally used alone.

Cocaine.—One part of the pure alkaloid dissolved in 2 parts of oleic acid.

Copper.—Ten and 20 per cent. ointments are generally used, the diluent being soft paraffin with a fifth of its weight of hard paraffin added to it. Lard is preferred by some physicians. Melt the oleate with the basis and stir until cold.

Iron.—Oleate and lard, equal parts.

Lead.—Hebra's ointment is a favourite remedy in skin diseases. It is generally made by melting lead plaster in its own weight of olive oil, but equal parts of the plaster and vaseline make a much better preparation. Melt the plaster first, then add the vaseline or oil, and perfume with oil of lavender.

Mercury.—Oleatum hydrargyri is an official preparation and contains 10 per cent. of mercuric oxide. Other strengths are 5 and 20 per cent., the former being liquid and the latter a stiff ointment. Oleates of mercury and morphine contain 1 grain of the alkaloid in each drachm, irrespective of the mercurial strength.

Nickel.—Oleate, 1 part ; lard, 7 parts.

Quinine.—One part of the alkaloid dissolved in 3 parts of oleic acid.

Silver.—One part of the oleate to 9 parts of lard.

Strychnine.—One part of the pure alkaloid dissolved in 3 parts of oleic acid.

Tin.—Oleate, 1 part ; lard or vaseline, 7 parts.

Veratrine.—1 grain dissolved in 50 minims of oleic acid.

Zinc.—The official 'oleatum' is an ointment. The powdered oleate is preferred in 25 per cent. ointment, with lard or vaseline as the diluent. The powder is largely used for dusting.

Lanoline is an admirable ointment basis, it being unoxidisable. It is sold in two forms, one with and one without contained water, which makes it white. Aqueous solutions are miscible with it to the extent of its own weight, so that if a soluble substance such as sulphate of zinc or cocaine hydrochlorate is to be made into an ointment with lanoline it should first be dissolved in as small a quantity of water as possible and mixed with the cold lanoline. The base should not, as a rule, be melted.

Mercurial Ointments.—A series of experiments published in *The Chemist and Druggist* some years ago go to prove that mercurial ointments may be made with steel knives with impunity, unless an acid or aqueous ingredient be present. Opodeldoc with ung. hydrarg. in equal proportions is sometimes prescribed in Germany. It is impossible so to combine these that they shall remain mixed. The only method of producing from them a permanent ointment is to rub down the ingredients of the opodeldoc, the camphor with a little spirit, the soap-powder, the essential oils, and sufficient spirit to dissolve them, and employ so much more lard instead of spirit.

Paraffin Ointments.—The ointments made with the new B.P. basis (a mixture of hard and soft paraffins) are apt to be granular unless they are very carefully made. Melt the paraffins over a water-bath, pour into a mortar previously well warmed with boiling water, and stir *constantly* until cold. If the ointment contain any powder, rub this up with a little of the soft paraffin before adding the melted mixture.

Perchloride of Mercury and Iodide of Potassium.—When these salts are prescribed together in an ointment, rub them in a mortar until perfectly smooth, then add the fatty matter.

Thymol should only be combined in a state of solution. The best way of doing this is to add about its own weight of camphor and rub them together. These form an amorphous fluid. Crystals of thymol are exceedingly irritating.

Order of Mixing is sometimes as important in the case of ointments as in mixtures, *e.g.* :—

Liq. antim. terchlor.	.	.	.	.	♏ v.
Hydrarg. ammon. chlor.	.	.	.	.	gr. xx.
Hydrarg. nit. ox.	.	.	.	.	gr. xv.
Potassæ subcarb.	.	.	.	.	℥j.
Adipis .	.	.	.	.	℥j.

This ointment retains its pink colour if the carbonate of potash be rubbed down with a little lard, but if dissolved in a few drops of water, the final addition of the liq. antim. terchlor. produces a brown colour, due to the formation of ferric hydrate, iron always occurring in commercial samples of 'butter of antimony.' In a fatty medium the incompatibles are slow to react. This is further instanced by the fact that tannin ointments may with impunity be made with a steel spatula, as no blackening occurs unless an aqueous ingredient is present.

Sending out Ointments.—If the patient can afford it, always send out ointments in covered pots. If not use chip boxes, preferably flat shape, previously dipped in melted hard paraffin ; it is customary to cover with 'waxed paper.' Preference should be given to paraffined paper : wax or stearine paper is often rancid, and affects the ointment.

PLASTERS.

IT is seldom nowadays that the dispenser is called upon to spread other than a cantharides plaster, and, consequently, few of the rising generation can handle the plaster-spatula with average dexterity. Of course emp. lyttæ is spread with the thumb ; it is generally spread on adhesive plaster on moleskin, so that an adhesive margin is provided. Some dispensers have a curious objection to use paper shapes ; there is no good reason why these should not be employed. If a shape be not used, a portion of plaster may be worked into a pencil-like roll, with which to form a border, afterwards filling-in in the ordinary manner. Other plasters are spread with the plaster-spatula. There should be no hesitation about the way to melt the plaster. Sufficient for the surface required is shaved off the roll and melted in a porcelain dish over a gentle gas-flame or water-bath. This in the long run is the safest and surest plan. While the plaster is melting the leather may be cut and prepared ; allow an inch all round for a margin. The shape of the plaster is cut from white wrapping paper, which should be wetted on the label-damper and placed on the margin. [Zinc shapes are kept for stock plasters.] By the time the paper shape is adjusted the plaster will have melted. The plaster must not be so hot as to frizzle up the leather, and the spatula, warmed in a gas-flame, should not cause the leather to curl. Having obtained the proper temperature (as low as will permit of easy spreading), the melted plaster is poured on the leather near the margin, the operator applies his spatula at a slight angle, the point of the blade slightly overlapping the paper shape. The plaster is pushed with a gently firm pressure in such a manner that the iron may not be raised from the leather until it has gone all round it (the leather being turned to suit the position of the operator, but the spreading must not be stopped while this is being done). Evenness of spreading is attained by regularity of pressure ; but no one can spread a plaster properly who does not do it in a few rapid strokes.

Paper Plaster Shapes may generally be attached to leather by merely damping the former, and pressing down with a dry cloth. If the shape is to be laid on a previously spread plaster, it should be well brushed with thin soft soap ; after its removal, any soap adhering to the plaster must be taken off with a wet cloth or sponge.

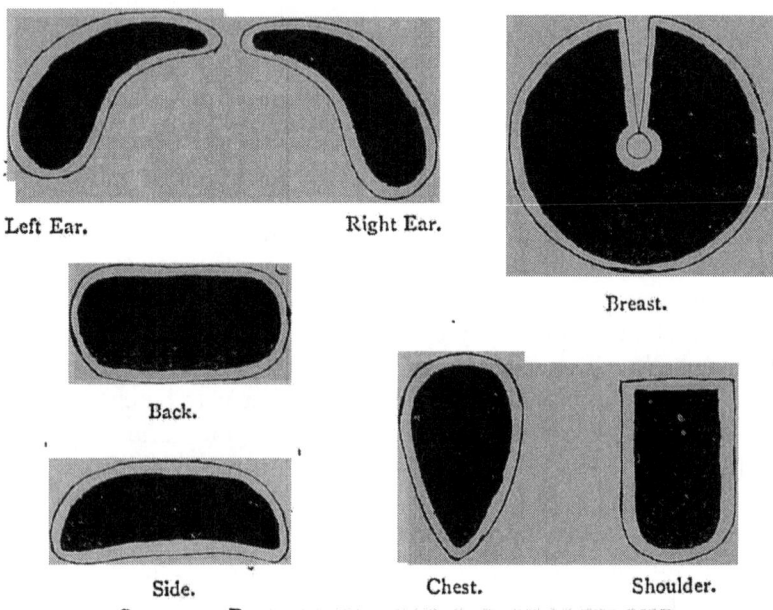

Left Ear.   Right Ear.

Breast.

Back.

Side.   Chest.   Shoulder.

SHAPES OF PLASTERS FOR DIFFERENT PARTS OF THE BODY.

Breast Plasters should be about 7 inches in diameter, exclusive of 1 inch margin, with a hole near the middle of 1 inch in diameter, and with a piece cut out, beginning from the hole and gradually widening towards the circumference to about 1 inch, so as to allow the plaster to be adapted to the curved surface of the breast.

Emp. canthar. should not be sprinkled with pulv. canthar.,

but a warm spatula used to smooth it. Some dispensers brush the surface with liquor epispasticus. This also is not admissible.

If a plaster is wanted soon after it is spread, place it on a cold metal surface, where it soon hardens. Waxed paper (or paper rubbed on one side with a piece of hard soap) should · be used for covering it. Send out in a box if possible.

JELLIES.

THE following comments by Hager on this class of preparations may be found useful :—

These, as medicinal vehicles, are prepared from various substances. For every 100 grammes of jelly are requisite 4 grammes of isinglass, 5 grammes of dry gelatine, 10 grammes carragheen, 15 grammes of Iceland moss, 10 grammes of starch, 10 grammes of hartshorn, 3 grammes of salep, or 5 grammes of tragacanth.

After boiling, skimming, &c., jellies should stand for three hours in a cold place. Medicinal additions should be made to the strained or skimmed jellies while hot.

Iceland-moss jellies need the addition of about 2 per cent. of isinglass or gelatine to impart the proper consistence and to keep their form. Generally, concentrated vegetable decoctions are added to clear jellies with one-tenth to one-fifth their weight of sugar during the boiling, and other additions, such as wine, medicinal syrups, &c., afterwards. Volatile oils are rubbed with sugar, and tinctures, bitter-almond water, &c., are added while the jellies are warm.

Jellies from fresh-fruit juices are made by combining the latter with half their weight of sugar, boiling and straining, skimming meanwhile. To 100 parts of juice, 1 part of isinglass or 2 parts of gelatine are added after skimming. The pectin in the juices forms, with the sugar, a gelatinising substance.

Copaiba, cod-liver oil, or castor-oil jellies are not jellies of the kind above described, but should rather be termed solidified fats (*e.g.*, *Oleum ricini solidificatum*). They are prepared by melting 5 or 6 parts of the oil or balsam with 1 part of sper-maceti, and leaving to cool. A cod-liver-oil jelly can be pre-pared from gelatine by the following process :—

Parts

Gelatine pure 20

Solve in
Aquæ fervidæ 150
Syrupi simplicis. 100

Tum adde
Olei jecoris aselli 250

(Olei anisi stellati gutt. 5)

Et agita in mortario lapideo, donec massam æquabilem præbeant, quæ semirefrigerata in vitrum infundatur ut loco frigido congelet.

MIXTURES.

THIS class of medicines is generally considered to require so little art in compounding, compared with the difficulty of reconciling a rebellious pill-mass, that certain principles which should be observed in preparing them are often overlooked by dispensers. Nearly all dispensing operations are more or less chemical ones. Dispensing is chemistry applied to the art of pharmacy ; but the skill and knowledge of the dispenser are generally most brought into request in letting as little chemical decomposition take place as possible. To such an extent do the disciples of Hahnemann carry this that a strict homœopath, in dosing a patient with aconite and belladonna, will make separate mixtures, containing only one of the tinctures in each, of which the patient must take a dose of one one hour, and of the other the next hour, and so on alternately.

In the introductory part of this treatise reference has been made to the various conditions which favour the production of uniform results. Everything else being equal, the dispenser should endeavour, in compounding mixtures or other solutions, to avoid chemical action as much as possible. Keep in mind that chemical action takes place more readily in presence of solvents than under any other condition. The one fundamental rule, therefore, in dispensing a physician's prescription is *to have as little chemical action take place among the ingredients of the formula as possible, unless such is clearly ordered or intended by the prescriber.* A typical mixture is like a quadruped—it has four legs to stand on. According to Pereira, these are the basis, the auxiliary (adjuvans), the corrective (corrigens), and the vehicle (excipiens) ; but as the tendency has of late been towards simplicity in prescribing, it frequently gets dismembered into a biped—either the auxiliary or the corrective, and, what is of more importance to the pocket of the pharmacist, the vehicle, are frequently omitted. The mixture is then, in pharmaceutical parlance, called 'drops.'

We shall best illustrate the difficulties in this department by giving examples of

TYPICAL MIXTURES.

In the following prescription gallic acid is present in excess of what the amount of water is capable of dissolving at the ordinary temperature :—

Acid. gallic.	ℨv.
Acid. sulph. dil.	℥j.
Aquæ	ad ℥viij.

Rub the gallic acid to a fine powder in a mortar, add the water and the sulphuric acid, and dispense with a 'shake the bottle' label. In this case the gallic acid dissolves with readiness in hot water, and some dispensers do follow this plan, but it is a very bad one, as the acid crystallises out on cooling. There are other substances, such as tannic acid, chlorate of potash, and quinine sulphate, with which a similar plan must be followed if sufficient solvent is not prescribed with them—viz. *rub to fine powder and mix with the vehicle.* It has been observed that chlorate of potash, when present in mixtures in excess, slowly becomes crystalline, due to changes in temperature.

It is always convenient, if there are no chemical reasons to prevent it, to take the ingredients of a formula, especially where these are numerous, in the order in which they are written, and use, weigh, or measure them out in this order. It is less tax on the memory to know when you have got so far among them that you have added all previously prescribed to the one being weighed or measured ; and the prescriber who has any knowledge of dispensing generally writes them in this order. The following is a good example of the value of this rule :—

Ol. santali flav.	.	.	.	.	.	.	℥ij.
Ol. copaibæ .	.	.	.	.	.	℈ss.
Tinc. cubebæ .	.	.	.	.	.	℥j.
Ol. menth. pip.	.	.	.	.	.	♏ xij.
Spt. vini rect. .	.	.	.	.	.	q.s. ut solve.
Tinct. buchu .	.	.	.	.	.	℥j.
Dec. Pareiræ .	.	.	.	.	.	℥v.
Inf. uvæ ursi .	.	.	.	.	.	℥v.

To compound in order as written is the best way possible
in such a case as this. Dissolve the first two oils in the tincture of cubebs, then the ol. menth. pip. in 2 drachms of
rectified spirit ; add this to the first solution, then the buchu
tincture, and gradually and with smart shaking the decoction
and infusion. If the latter are recently prepared, the mixture
is much more presentable than when made with concentrated
infusions.

To take another example, a prescription for a bronchitic
mixture which seems of no difficulty :—

Ammon. carb.	.	.	.	.	.	.	gr. 60
Syrupi tolutani	.	.	.	.	.	℥vj.
Tinct. tolutanæ	.	.	.	.	.	℥iij.
Vin. ipecac. .	.	.	.	.	.	℥ij.
Sp. chloroform.	.	.	.	.	.	℥iij.
Inf. senegæ	.	.	.	.	.	ad ℥xij.

Solve et misce.

Here the carbonate of ammonia must first be dissolved in the
infusion, and for that purpose a mortar will be required, as the
salt does not dissolve readily enough in aqueous menstrua to
enable us to make the solution in a measure-glass with the aid
of a glass rod, as might be done with bicarbonate of potash,
and in this case also shaking causes undesirable frothing.
Having got the solution of carbonate of ammonia in clear condition—say about a couple of ounces of it—in the bottle, syrup
of tolu comes second on the formula. But this should not be
added now, because it would clam up the measure, and we
should not be able to measure the other ingredients accurately
after it in the same glass, without cleaning it more than necessary for our present purpose. The ipecacuanha wine should

be added at this stage, but, before doing so, the solution should be diluted in the bottle with about 7 oz. more of the infusion. A word of caution about infusions. When freshly prepared they should be allowed to become quite cold before being used for dispensing. It is a common fault with dispensers not to do so, but if used warm in this instance it will partially volatilise the ammonia, chloroform, and some of the spirit, and cause the resin of tolu to deposit on the side of the bottle. Now mix the spirit of chloroform and tincture of tolu, and pour them into the bottle, being careful to let the liquid fall into the middle of the solution, and not touch the neck or side ; agitate the whole instantly by a little sudden jerking. In this way the resin and chloroform will be equally diffused through the mixture. On adding the spirit of chloroform by itself to such a mixture, without shaking, the chloroform would separate and descend, and on pouring in the tincture of tolu by itself, without shaking, the resin would separate and float on the top. By having the resin of tolu held in solution by the additional quantity of alcohol of the spirit of chloroform, less separation takes place on addition to the mixture. In other words, a better emulsion will be made of the resin than if the tincture had been poured in by itself. The syrup of tolu should now be added quickly, and the measure rinsed with more infusion —sufficient to make the required quantity of mixture. The bottle should be at last slightly—not too much—shaken, or it will have a tendency to make the resin separate on the sides of the bottle.

The rule in preparing these mixtures should be, therefore : Make a solution of the salts first, using the vehicle, which is generally aqueous, as a menstruum ; strain into the bottle, dilute with more vehicle passed through the strainer, add the tinctures, or spirits, measuring small quantities first, shaking after each addition ; then add the syrup or any mixed preparation ordered ; lastly fill up with the vehicle, and shake again. Sometimes syrup of squill is ordered in such a mixture as the foregoing. In this case, the dispenser should mix the carbonate solution with the syrup of squill before adding any other ingredient. If spirit of nitrous ether is also ordered, it should be separately neutralised with a small portion of the carbonate solution.

In the following another course requires to be adopted :—

Ammon. carb.	gr. vj.
Vin. ipecac.	ʒij.
Vin. antim.	ʒij.
Syr. scillæ	ʒiij.
Syr. mori	ʒiv.
Aquæ	ad ℥iss.

There is so little aqueous menstruum here that, if the usual course is adopted, effervescence is most persistent, and it may be an hour before it entirely subsides. Powder the carbonate and, in place of adding the syrup of squill, take a proportionate quantity of acetum scillæ—viz. 78 minims. When the effervescence has ceased, which is almost immediately, transfer the solution to the bottle, add the vin. ipec., vin. antim., and syr. mori, and make up to 1½ oz. with simple syrup.

Another example is a mixture containing insoluble salts with tragacanth to suspend them. The great object in this is to give the patient in each dose of the mixture an equal quantity of each ingredient, having the solids suspended in it with the aid of the gums in the state of fine powder.

Bismuth. subnit.	ʒij.
Magnes. carb.	ʒj.
Acid. hydrocyan. (Scheele) . . .	♏ vj.
Tr. capsici	♏ x.
Tr. opii	fl. ʒiss.
Pulv. tragac. co.	ʒiss.
Aq. menth. pip.	ad fl. ℥vj.

Mix.

The three powders require rubbing together in a mortar, with some of the vehicle gradually poured in to form a uniform mixture; this should be transferred to the bottle, the liquids added (the acid last) in the bottle, *not the mortar*, else loss by evaporation of hydrocyanic acid will take place. The mortar should be rinsed with a little more of the vehicle, this poured into the bottle, and the quantity required to fill the bottle added. Not infrequently dispensers put powders, such as bismuth and magnesia, into a bottle, and pour mucilage directly upon them, the result being that the powders are diffused in a lumpy condition. Powders ought always to be mixed with water before adding mucilage.

We remember a candidate at the minor examination, who had a mixture containing powdered rhubarb and bicarbonate of soda to dispense, giving in the mixture with the rhubarb floating on the surface! Had he carefully mixed the powders with water before pouring into the bottle this would not have happened.

When fluids are to be mixed which decompose each other, or may form combinations, the order of mixing may have a considerable influence on the condition and appearance of the mixture. Example :—

Liquor. ferri perchlor.	. . . . .	꒞ij.
Mucil. acaciæ	. . . . .	꒞j.
Aquæ destillatæ	. . . . .	ad ꒞viij.

If the mucilage be added to the iron solution the two form a gelatinous mass, which will not make a clear solution with the rest of the water. But a clear yellow fluid is obtained if the iron and the mucilage are each first diluted with half of the water and then mixed, or if the iron is mixed with all the water and the mucilage added last.

So, also, when tannin fluids have to be mixed with metallic salts or alkaloids. In such cases both should be well diluted before combination. Example :—

Plumbi acetatis	. . . . .	꒞j.
Tincturæ opii	. . . . .	꒞ij.
Syrupi	. . . . .	꒞vj.
Aquæ	. . . . .	ad ꒞viij.

In this case the acetate of lead should be dissolved in ꒞iv. of water, and the tincture of opium diluted with the rest of the water and added to the solution. In this way a slightly cloudy mixture is obtained, instead of a mixture with insoluble flakes floating in it.

When vegetable substances, wholly or partially soluble in water, especially such as contain tannin or like constituents, have to be mixed with metallic or earthy salts, the rule is that both the vegetable and the salt should be first dissolved in a large portion of the water and mixed. If a precipitate is formed it is then easily diffused by shaking.

The following is a favourite recipe with a West-End physician :—

Liq. ferri dialy. (Wyeth)	℥iv.
Liq. arsenicalis.	℥ss.
Aq. dest.	ad ℥vj.

If the old-fashioned plan of 'putting everything in first and then filling up' be followed, a thick mixture will result. If, however, the dialysed iron be *well* diluted with the water before adding the Fowler's solution, a beautifully bright mixture can be made.

These examples sufficiently illustrate the importance of carefully considering the order of mixing ; it is useful to note the following : *First*, that where either syrup, glycerine, honey, or mucilage is ordered along with fluids which decompose each other or which produce unsightly combinations, it is highly probable the prescriber has foreseen and anticipated this result, and has added this particular ingredient to avoid or mitigate the evil. Glycerine has in many cases a powerful influence in preventing decompositions, as well as in preventing depositions ; syrup, less so ; while honey and mucilage are favourable to fine division and suspension of insoluble salts and organic matter. *Second*, that where any decomposition takes place producing unsightly mixtures, as in the case of resinous solutions and extracts, or where a homogeneous mixture generally is desired, a much better result will be obtained by using the mortar and pestle, as in the production of an emulsion, than by agitating the ingredients in a bottle. *Lastly*, in no case should liberties be permitted in the shape of additions to or subtractions from prescriptions, with a view to producing what is called 'elegant pharmacy.' Cases where such expedients are necessary are very rare, and even in these the error is generally obviously due to the neglect or oversight of the pre-scriber, and is so apparent that the dispenser cannot possibly have any difficulty in the matter

CHEMICAL CHANGES.

A common case of chemical incompatibility is in prescriptions such as the following, containing potassium iodide and spirit of nitrous ether :—

Potassæ bitart.	ʒj.
Potassii iodidi	ʒj.
Spt. ætheris nitrosi	ʒiv.
Syr. aurantii	ʒj.
Aquæ	ad ʒx.

This mixture cannot be dispensed without reaction between the potassium bitartrate and iodide and spirit of nitrous ether, iodine and nitrous oxide being liberated, thus :—

$$KHC_4H_4O_6 + C_2H_5NO_2 + KI = K_2C_4H_4O_6 + C_2H_5HO + NO + I.$$

If the dispenser can communicate with the prescriber, he should inform him that the mixture will contain free iodine, and also that it will not contain a particle of nitrous ether ; if he cannot be consulted, proceed as follows: Dissolve 1 drachm of cream of tartar and 8 grains of potassium iodide in 4 oz. of water contained in a mortar, add the spirit of nitrous ether, stir briskly, so that the gas may escape, and allow to stand for half an hour in order to get rid of the nitrous fumes entirely. Then make up the rest of the mixture and add it to the contents of the mortar. The object of this procedure is to limit the action of the nitrous ether, for while theoretically the 4 drachms will liberate the iodine from about 8 grains only of iodide, the liberated nitrous oxide on coming in contact with air is changed to higher oxides, which are capable of decomposing iodide, so that if the mixture were made up in a 10-oz. bottle, iodine would continue to be liberated, until the whole of the iodide of potassium was decomposed.

It frequently happens that chemical changes take place in

mixtures which are quite unanticipated by both prescriber and dispenser. In the following, apart from separation of sulphate of magnesia in crystals, owing to the presence of so large an amount of spirit, the mixture gradually acquires a bluish colour :—

Ammon. brom.	ʒiij.
Tinct. nucis vom.	ʒiv.
Sp. chloroformi	ʒiij.
Magnes. sulph.	ʒss.
Sp. ammon. co.	ʒiv.
Syr. zingib.	ʒj.
Aq. menth. pip.	ad ʒvj.

It takes some time before this colour is developed, and it appears to be due to reaction between the igasuric acid of the nux vomica and the alkali in the mixture. It also occurs in mixtures of liquor bismuthi and tincture of nux. A somewhat analogous change takes place in the following mixture :—

Pot. bicarb.	ʒij.
Sodæ salicyl.	ʒiss.
Vin. colchici	ʒiv.
Aquæ	ad ʒviij.

This assumes a colour almost like compound tincture of cardamoms after standing forty-eight hours. It is a matter of common observation that aqueous solutions of alkaline salicylates become of a reddish-brown colour on exposure to light, apparently due to the oxidation products of salicylic acid being accompanied by coloured bodies. Stock solution of the bicarbonate induces the coloration more readily than the bicarbonate itself, owing to the solution containing carbonate. Natural salicylic acid is not so liable to change.

Tincture of nux vomica, owing to the alkaloids which it contains, is very apt to change colour when mixed with nitric acid or nitro-muriatic acid. For instance—

Acid. nitrici dil.	ʒiv.
Aquæ destillat.	ʒvj.
Tinct. nucis vomicæ .	ʒij.

If mixed in the order written, the mixture soon becomes yellow-coloured and acquires an odour of nitrous acid ; if the order be reversed, neither colour nor odour is developed. Various results are produced by mixing part of the water with the acid and part with the tincture. A red or reddish-yellow colour develops in course of time, but is ultimately discharged. This applies more particularly to acid. nitro-mur. dil. and nux vomica mixtures.

MIXTURES BECOMING GELATINOUS.

We have already referred to the fact that some kinds of distilled water become perfectly gelatinous on keeping. The same thing takes place with some kinds of mixtures. The following are cases which have been observed by correspondents of *The Chemist and Druggist* :—

Tinct. hamamelis	♏ 40
Ext. ergotæ liq.	ʒj.
Spt. æther. chlor.	ʒj.
Syr. papav. alb.	ʒij.
Tr. nuc. vom.	♏ 40
Aquæ	ad ℥viij.

Two days after this mixture was dispensed it was returned a perfectly gelatinous mass. It had every appearance of a perfect mixture when sent out, and remained so about twelve hours, when it changed in colour from almost transparent brown to opaque pink, and became thick and ropy. A mixture containing syr. pap. alb. and syr. scillæ became ropy and of a pink colour when made with old syr. papav., but when made with fresh syrup it kept all right. Sulphate of quinine, tinct. ferri perchlor. and spt. chloroform. with water sometimes form a mixture resembling calf's-foot jelly.

The following mixture becomes a glutinous-looking product after it has been made, say, thirty-six hours :—

Ferri et ammon. cit.	gr. 80
Aquæ	℥iv.
Syr. aurant.	℥j.
Sol. nitroglycerini, 1 per cent.	♏ xvj.
Aquæ	ad ℥viij.

All these cases are of great interest. The change to the gelatinous condition appears to be due to the presence of the organism known as the viscous ferment, the cells of which form thread-like groups which ramify through the fluid and make it gelatinous, just as fibrin does in the case of coagulated blood. The development of the organism appears to be due to the presence of nitrogenous bodies—for example, in the last prescription the solution of nitro-glycerine is probably the cause. The dispenser cannot possibly know when a mixture will become viscous; it may become so at one time and not at another. All that he can do is to explain the matter when it does happen, and in nine cases out of ten customers will be satisfied with the explanation. It is useful to note that the presence of a good proportion of alcohol—say 20 per cent.—prevents the change.

There are several **Protective Fluids,** the presence of which may prevent a precipitate or retard a chemical change in a mixture. The more important members of the group are glycerine, syrup, and mucilage. The method employed is to dissolve any tincture likely to separate in an aqueous menstruum in one of these first, if present in the recipe. Thus, in the case of the lead and opium mixture mentioned before, dispense the prescription as follows :—

Dissolve plumbi acet., Əj., in | Tinct. opii, ʒij.
Aq. dest., ʒvj. | Syrupi simpl., ʒvj.
 | Aquæ, ʒiss.

Mix the two solutions.

The tincture of opium does not escape separation so much from being diluted as on account of being *protected*. Preparations of cinchona, gum-resins, and numerous others follow the same rule. Ext. cinchon. liq. is frequently prescribed in mixtures along with glycerine : of course, mix the extract with the glycerine before diluting.

CASES WHERE CHEMICAL ACTION IS INTENDED.

Saline Mixtures.—In many cases there is clearly a chemical action intended, as in the case of saline mixtures, which are extemporaneously prepared solutions of the alkaline acetates, citrates, etc. For example :—

Potass. bicarb.	℥ij.
Ammon. carb.	℥ss.
Acid. citric.	℥ij.
Syrup.	℥ss.
Aq.	ad ℥vj.

Here the prescriber intends the mixture to contain carbonic acid gas in solution, and, to obtain this, after powdering the carbonate of ammonia the bicarbonate of potash should be added to it in the mortar, then the acid with a little water (but *not the syrup*), the effervescence allowed to pass off and the solution strained, the syrup added *in the bottle*, and the quantity made up and quickly corked. The mixture will not effervesce, but it will have the fresh taste of the little free carbonic acid it contains.

Effervescing Mixtures distinct from the foregoing are frequently ordered by medical men, the usual method being to prescribe an alkaline mixture and acid powders, although there are cases in which an alkaline and an acid mixture are sent out together. It is important that the directions should be quite distinct. It frequently occurs, also, that the prescriber, probably forgetful of his saturation tables, leaves the dose of acid to the discretion of the dispenser ; if this should occur the dispenser may put in a slight excess of acid—it improves the taste in most cases. The following are examples of this class of mixture :—

Ferri et ammon. cit.	℥j.
Acid. citric.	℥ij.
Aquæ	ad ℥vj.

M. Sig. : No 1.

Potass. bicarb. .   .   .   . ℥iij

Syr. limonis   .   .   .   . ℥j.

Aquæ   .   .   .   . ad ℥xij.

M. Sig. : No. 2.

One tablespoonful of No. 1 to be taken with two tablespoonfuls of No. 2 twice a day, etc.

It may appear that the prescriber has erred in placing the syrup of lemon in the alkaline mixture, thereby neutralising it, but it will be observed that there remains after the doses are mixed a slight excess of citric acid—viz. $1\frac{1}{2}$ grain in each dose.

Sodæ tartaratæ   .   .   .   .   .   . ℥vj.

Sodæ bicarb. .   .   .   . ℥iij.

Vin. antim.   .   .   .   .   .   . ℥iss.

Syr. aurant.   .   .   .   .   .   . ℥j.

Aquæ   .   .   .   .   .   . ad ℥viij.

Sig. : ℥j. 4tis h. ex. aq.

Pulv. acid. tart.   .   .   .   .   .   . q.s. [20 grs.]

Tales viij.

Sig. : j. with each dose of the medicine.

The directions require slight modification, and the dispenser is quite within his province if he puts on the bottle some such label as this : 'Two tablespoonfuls (by measure-glass) every four hours, in water. Add one of the powders, and drink during effervescence.'

The dispenser must also rely on his own knowledge for the quantity of acid to be sent in each powder, or he may refer to the following table compiled by Prof. Attfield, F.R.S.

SATURATION TABLES.

In round numbers, for purposes of prescribing and dispensing.

Acidum citricum	20	19	17	14	10	17	24	30
Acidum tartaricum	22	20	18	15	11	18	26	32
Potassæ carbonas	24	22	20	16	12	20	28	35
Potassæ bicarbonas	29	27	24	20	14	24	34	42
Sodæ carbonas	40	38	35	28	20	34	49	60
Sodæ bicarbonas	24	22	20	17	12	20	29	36
Ammoniæ carbonas	17	16	14	12	8	14	20	25
Magnesiæ carbonas	14	13	11	9	7	11	16	20

The table is read thus : 20 grains of citric acid will saturate 29 grains of bicarbonate of potassium ; 20 grains of bicarbonate of sodium will saturate, or be saturated by, 18 grains of tartaric acid ; 11 grains of tartaric acid = 8 grains of carbonate of ammonium ; 20 grains of bicarbonate of sodium are equivalent to, or will do as much work as, 34 grains of carbonate of sodium ; 14 grains of citric acid are as strong as 15 grains of tartaric acid. It is occasionally convenient to double the numbers, halve them, or take some other proportion ; also to employ them in weights other than grains.

Lemon-juice contains, on an average, $32\frac{1}{2}$ grains of citric acid in 1 fl. oz., or 4 grains per fl. drachm.

Chlorinated Solutions.—A prescription which seems to turn up periodically, even in the examination-room, is for chlorate of potassium, hydrochloric acid, and water. The mixture is used for scarlatina, and other disorders in which the throat is affected. The object is to make a solution of chlorine ; and this is done by adding the acid direct to the salt, corking the bottle for a short time, and then adding the water.

The prescription is a revived form of a very old recipe invented by the late Mr. Beamish, of Covent Garden. He gained some reputation for the formula, which was intended to be a specific in case of hay-fever. It was as follows :—

Sodii chlorid.	ʒij.
Potass. chlorat.	ʒij.
Acid. hydrochl. pur.	ʒiv.
Aquæ destillat.	ad ℥ij.

M. Ft. guttæ secund. art. Minim doses only in water.

The chlorine is likewise liberated in a dilute solution, but, of course, more gradually, and for this reason some pharmacists are of the opinion that it is not always intended that the acid should be added to the chlorate, but that chlorine should be slowly liberated. This idea is, however, very ridiculous when one bears in mind that the mixture must become chlorinated at some time, and it is better that this should be before it reaches the patient's hands.

QUININE MIXTURES.

QUININE SALTS give rise to so many curious complications when dispensed in mixture form that some special remarks are necessary regarding them. As to the solution of quinine in acids, the fact that the mineral acids, strong or dilute, make presentable pill-masses indicates that they should not be poured direct upon a quinine salt, but that the salt should be well diffused in water before the acid is added. Very often, however, no acid is ordered in the prescription. In such a case it is extremely unwise to depart from the letter of the physician's order. The only admissible manner of compounding is to reduce the quinine salt to fine powder, and diffuse it in the liquids. In some cases, as when spirit of ether is an ingredient, the quinine tends to adhere to the bottle, but this may be avoided by the addition of a little mucilage of acacia to the mixture. Some dispensers advocate that the quinine should be dissolved in such circumstances, and the view is one for which there is much to be said; but quinine in solution is much more bitter than when in suspension, and this fact throws the balance of opinion in favour of the suspension method.

The greater number of difficulties with quinine mixtures occur through the precipitation of the quinine after it has been brought into solution. The simplest of these, apart from those due to ordinary alkaloidal precipitants, are caused by the formation of less soluble salts owing to double decomposition— for example, in the case of mindererus spirit and a solution of sulphate of quinine. It so happens that acetate of quinine is one of its least soluble salts, although it dissolves readily on heating, and in certain proportions it is possible to get a mixture of an alkaline acetate and quinine sulphate perfectly solid owing to the formation of quinine acetate. Salicylates also form sparingly soluble compounds with soluble quinine salts.

The most unmanageable mixtures are those in which are alkaloidal precipitants. The more common of these which are found associated with quinine in prescriptions are the alkaline carbonates and hydrates, iodides and iodine, perchloride of mercury, and infusions or tinctures containing tannin. In all circumstances these substances precipitate quinine as insoluble compounds which in most cases are adhesive. The alkaline hydrates and carbonates precipitate quinine as hydrate, and there is no means of avoiding the precipitation. Prescribers appear to be fonder of ordering the alkalies—generally in the form of aromatic spirit of ammonia—with citrate of iron and quinine than with the plain salts of quinine, probably under the impression that the double salt is not affected by the alkali. Ammoniated tincture of quinine also is sometimes prescribed along with water, the result being that quinine hydrate is precipitated, the alkaloid existing in the tincture in that form being kept in solution by the alcohol. Examples of such cases are given in the following pages, and it will be seen that the addition of mucilage is recommended, this being all that is necessary to diffuse the precipitated quinine permanently in the mixture instead of letting it adhere to the bottle.

Iodide of potassium forms different compounds with quinine salts, the difference depending upon the other ingredients of the mixture. Neutral solutions of quinine sulphate and potassium iodide do not react chemically, but the presence of free acid invariably induces a chemical change, and this is accentuated if there is any substance in the mixture which liberates iodine, such as nitric acid or spirits of nitre. Once an alkaloid in solution comes into contact with free iodine all hope of a satisfactory mixture is gone. In such cases the dispenser should, if possible, communicate with the prescriber, so as to suggest the exclusion of the oxidising body; failing that, the reaction between the alkaline iodide and the oxidising body should be carried out with the minimum quantity of iodide, the rest of the iodide being mixed with the quinine and a little mucilage before the iodine solution is added to it. Double iodides, such as *liquor arsenii et hydrargyri iodidi* (Donovan's solution), precipitate alkaloids at once; the same is the case with perchloride of mercury, the precipitates being heavy and therefore dangerous. Galenical preparations containing tannin, especially the acid infusion of roses, are troublesome when prescribed along with quinine salts, and require special treatment.

Other difficulties of a similar nature occasionally occur, but most of them are amenable to the two rules which should be observed—viz. :—

1. Chemical reaction should be effected in the most dilute solutions; and
2. A means for the proper apportioning of the dose should be adopted. For this purpose mucilage of acacia is not only generally suitable, but it has been shown to retard or modify chemical action.

We now give a number of prescriptions which have actually been met with at the dispensing-counter.

With Carbonates or Hydrates quinine frequently forms a troublesome precipitate which requires careful management. The best result is usually obtained by diluting, as far as possible, the incompatible solutions *before* mixing. This method answers with the following :—

Tinct. quininæ	℥j.
Ammon. carb.	℥j.
Aq.	ad ℥xij.

But if the tincture be poured into a strong solution of the carbonate, the alkaloid separates in flocks, which adhere to the sides of the bottle.

Quininæ sulph.	℈ij.
Sp. ammon. ar.	℥vj.
Aq.	ad ℥vj.

Mixed in whatever manner, the precipitated quinine adheres in lumps. A good mixture was, however, obtained by using a proportionate quantity of pure quinine instead of sulphate ; this was diffused through a portion of the water, and the diluted sal volatile added.

Quininæ sulph.	.	.	.	.	.	gr. xvj.
Sp. œtheris .	.	.	.	.	.	ʒij.
Sp. ammon. ar.	.	.	.	.	.	ʒiv.
Tr. opii	.	.	.	.	.	♏ xxx.
Aquæ .	.	.	.	.	.	ad ʒviij.

The plan to follow in this case is to rub the quinine to fine powder in a mortar, and mix it with 7 oz. of water. Add the sal volatile, shake well, then add the rest of the ingredients and sufficient water to make up to 8 oz. In this case the alkaline spirit would decompose the quinine sulphate, and this decomposition is brought down to a minimum by the method described.

With Bicarbonates. —When these are ordered with quinine in a prescription, the bicarbonate should be dissolved in the water, and the quinine rubbed to a fine powder and suspended in the liquid. The addition of a little mucilage has the effect in these cases of suspending the quinine and preventing it from adhering to the sides of the bottle.

With Iodides. —Prescriptions containing quinine sulphate and potassium iodide are not uncommon. Dissolve the sulphate of quinine with as little acid as possible, and separately dissolve the potassium iodide in about four times its weight of water, dilute the quinine solution and add the iodide to it.

Liq. ferri iodidi .	.	.	.	.	.	ʒss.
Syr. ferri hypophosph.	.	.	.	.	.	ʒj.
Quininæ phosph.	.	.	.	.	.	ʒij.
Acid. phosph. dil.	.	.	.	.	.	ʒss.

The liquor added to a solution of the quinine in the acid gives a copious finely divided precipitate of 'quinine iodide,' but if the syrup be added *before* the liquor, a clear solution is obtained, from which the quinine iodide gradually crystallises. The former method should be adopted.

The amount of acid used to dissolve the quinine exerts a

certain influence on the nature of the precipitate formed. For example, in the case of the following :—

Quininæ sulphatis .	.	.	.	.	.	gr. xxiv.
Acid. nitric. dil. .	.	.	.	.	.	q. s.
Potassii iodidi	.	.	.	.	.	ʒij.
Aquæ .	.	.	.	.	.	ad ℥vj.

Here use just sufficient dilute acid, ♏25, to dissolve the quinine, and a yellow precipitate of iodide of quinine is formed; but if a large excess of acid be added it liberates iodine from the potassium iodide, and the liberated iodine combines with the sulphate of quinine to form the insoluble iodosulphate of quinine, or herapathite, which is gradually deposited as a greenish-brown sediment.

In some cases of this kind it is not herapathite which is formed, but a brown compound of sulphate of quinine, iodide of quinine, and iodine. This is more especially the case with mixtures containing quinine sulphate, potassium iodide, and spirit of nitrous ether, such as the following :—

Quininæ sulph.	.	.	.	.	.	gr. xxx.
Potassii iodid.	.	.	.	.	.	gr. xx.
Sp. ammon. ar.	.	.	.	.	.	ʒvj.
Sp. æther. nit.	.	.	.	.	.	ʒiv.
Tinct. zingib.	.	.	.	.	.	ʒiij.
Aq.	.	.	.	.	.	ad ℥vj.

Numerous futile attempts were made to combine this in a presentable manner; the prescriber being near, he was consulted, and direction was given to dispense the iodide and sal volatile in a separate mixture.

The bromides form perfectly clear mixtures with quinine. The following gives a clear mixture, the hydrobromate being a soluble salt :—

Quininæ bromidi	.	.	.	.	.	ʒij.
Acid. hydrobromici (medic.)	.	.	.	.	ʒiij.
Spt. ætheris chlorici .	.	.	.	.	ʒvj.
Tinc. lavand. co.	.	.	.	.	.	ʒj.
Aq. destillat. .	.	.	.	.	.	ad ℥viij.

Dissolve the quinine hydrobromate in 4 oz. of water, and add to it the chloric ether. Mix the tincture, acid, and 2 oz.

of water together and filter into the quinine solution, if an absolutely clear mixture is desired.

With Tannin.—We have already remarked that tannin precipitates alkaloids. Here is a good instance :—

Quininæ sulph.	.	.	.	.	.	. gr. ix.
Acid. sulph. dil.	.	.	.	.	.	. ʒij.
Infus. rosæ	.	.	.	.	.	ad ℥viij.

The formation of an insoluble tannate of quinine cannot be avoided. Sometimes a dispenser expecting to obtain a perfectly transparent mixture, and surprised at the result, is disposed to filter out the tannate of quinine. This, of course, is unjustifiable, as is every other attempt to remove a thera- peutically active precipitate in any mixture.

With Salicylates quinine sulphate forms a precipitate of salicylate of quinine. The two following are good examples :—

Lithiæ salicylat.	.	.	.	.	.	ʒij.
Potass. iodid.	.	.	.	.	.	ʒss.
Ferri et quininæ cit.	.	.	.	.	.	ʒj.
Aq. chloroformi	.	.	.	.	.	ad ℥viij.

In this case dissolve the citrate in an ounce of chloroform water, and the salicylate and iodide in the rest contained in a measure or mortar, then add the citrate solution gradually to it, stirring assiduously in order to break up the precipitate thoroughly. The mixture is a bad one, however prepared.

Quininæ sulph.	.	.	.	.	.	. gr. xx.
Sodii salicylat.	.	.	.	.	.	. ℥ss.
Acid. hydrobromici	.	.	.	.	.	. ʒj.
Aquæ	.	.	.	.	.	. ad ℥viij.

The hydrobromic acid acts on the salicylate of soda, pre- cipitating salicylic acid. Salicylate of quinine is also formed if the quinine has been dissolved with the acid. The following is a good method of procedure : Dissolve 90 grains of the salicylate in 4 oz. of water in a mortar, and to this add the hydrobromic acid gradually, stirring constantly. Rub the quinine to fine powder, mix an ounce of water with it, dissolve the rest of the salicylate in 2 oz. of water, and add to the mixture in the mortar.

Sodæ salicylat. .	ʒj.
Tinct. quininæ .	ʒvj.
Aquæ	ad ʒvj.

In this case also a precipitate of salicylate of quinine is formed which is not dissolved by the addition of acids.

With Liquorice Extract.—This extract is well known as an excellent covering for the taste of quinine ; consequently we occasionally find the two together in mixture, with far from good results.   Thus:—

Ferri et quininæ citratis .	ʒiss.
Ammonii chloridi	ʒij.
Ext. glycyrrhizæ liq.	ʒss.
Aquæ	ad ʒiv.

In this mixture a dense precipitate is formed which renders it most unsightly.   So also in the following :—

Sodii sulph. .	ʒj.
Quininæ sulph.	gr. xx.
Acid. sulph. dil.	ʒij.
Ext. glycyrrhizæ liq.	ʒvj.
Aquæ	ad ʒviij.

However dispensed a precipitate is unavoidable.   Compounded as written a thick flaky precipitate is produced, which, when allowed to stand for a day, becomes tenacious and hardly diffusible.   Omitting the acid, the precipitate is very fine and easily diffused through the liquid.   The explanation is that liquorice extract is very readily decomposed by alkaloidal solutions, with separation of *glycyrrhizin*, the sweet principle of liquorice.   There are several inorganic salts which precipitate the glycyrrhizin, as, for example, sodium sulphate and potassium acid tartrate.   In the second prescription the acid also has an influence in inducing separation, less of it giving a better-looking mixture.

Tr. Quininæ Ammon. is a preparation in which the quinine exists as hydrate, kept in solution by means of the excess of ammonia, and by the rectified spirit, more especially the latter. Consequently when it is mixed with much water the alkaloid is precipitated, as in the following :—

Tr. quininæ ammoniatæ .	. . . . .	3x.
Ammon. bromid. .	. . . . .	3iss.
Syr. aurantii .	. . . . .	℥ss.
Aq. camph. .	. . . . .	ad ℥vj.

Science cannot prevent the precipitation without inducing chemical change. The addition of a few drachms of mucilage would suspend the quinine equally throughout the mixture.

Or you may take an equivalent quantity of quinine sulphate, rub it up with the bromide to a very fine powder, add the syrup, water, and spirit, and the ammonia solution last.

SCALE PREPARATIONS IN MIXTURES.

Scale preparations are not difficult of solution, tartarated iron and sulphate of beberine being the most difficult to dissolve. Do not shake scale preparations with a solvent, as an abundant and persistent froth is in most cases formed. We subjoin examples of mixtures containing scale preparations, which will show the difficulties which may arise and how to deal with them.

Ferri et quininæ cit. .	. . . . .	gr. xxxvj.
Sp. ammon. arom. .	. . . .	3iij.
Syr. zingiberis .	. . . .	3ij.
Aq. .	. . . . .	ad ℥vj.

Dissolve the ferri et quininæ cit. in 2 oz. of water, and the other ingredients in the remainder ; mix with gentle agitation.

Ferri am. cit.	. . . . . .	3j.
Acid. cit. .	. . . . . .	3j.
Tinct. aurant. .	. . . . .	℥iij.
Syr. aurant.	. . . . . .	3j.

The solution of the ferri am. cit. is troublesome ; it should be dissolved in a test-tube, with a drachm of water, over a spirit-lamp. If the mixture is not wanted immediately the ammonio-citrate will dissolve if added last to the other ingredients contained in the bottle, this being laid on its side ; with an occa-

L

sional shake, in less than half an hour it will be dissolved.
Ferri et quin. cit. is sometimes prescribed in this form, and the
same procedure is to be adopted.

Ferri et ammonii citras, with potassium or sodium bicarbonate, in solution, always effervesces. When ordered together
in a mixture the cork should be left out for a time to allow the
carbonic acid gas to escape.

Ferri et quininæ cit.	ℨj.
Potass. citrat.	ℨiv.
Syr. aurant.	℥ss.
Aq.	ad ℥vj.

Even with perfectly neutral citrate of potash there is a considerable deposit of quinine in this mixture. This appears to
be due to the excess of acid in the ferri et quin. cit. combining
with the potash salt to form an acid citrate whereby the quinine
citrate is allowed to drop out of solution. The addition of a
few grains of citric acid forms a perfectly clear mixture.

Tincturæ digitalis	ℨj.
Ferri et quininæ citratis	ℨij.
Acidi phosphorici diluti	ℨj.
Infusi quassiæ	ad ℥vj.

If compounded in the order of the ingredients—*i.e.* the citrate
being dissolved in a little of the infusion—the tincture precipitates a little of the quinine as tannate, and the phosphoric acid
throws out a portion of the iron as phosphate.

Tannic acid, perchloride of mercury, iodide of potassium,
carbonates, and bicarbonates all precipitate alkaloids. The
last prescription quoted shows how the little tannin in tincture
of digitalis has this effect. In the following case we have a
more flagrant example of incompatibility :—

Ferri et quin. cit.	ℨj.
Ammon. carb.	ℨij.
Tinct. aurant. . . . . . ;	℥ij.
Aq.	ad ℥vj.

No plan can be adopted for preventing the precipitation of
the quinine in this case. The best results are obtainable by

dissolving the citrate in ℥ss. of water, and mixing it with the tincture. Dissolve the ammonia in the remainder of the water and mix the two solutions, pouring the citrate solution into the ammonia one. The addition of a little mucilage to the ammonia solution before mixing would prevent the quinine adhering to the bottle, and the dispenser should not hesitate to add it.

Bromide of potassium upsets the equilibrium of ferrum tartaratum.

Ferri tartarat.	ℨj.
Potassii brom.	ℨiij.
Tinct. chlorof. co.	ℨivss.
Syr. zingib.	ℨvj.
Aq. menthæ pip.	ad ℥vj.

The tartrate must be dissolved separately by rubbing down to powder in a mortar and stirring with 3 oz. of the peppermint-water. By attempting to dissolve it along with the bromide an insoluble coating is formed on its surface, and solution is very much retarded.

Sulphate of beberine should have a little dilute sulphuric acid added to it, as well as hot water. The solution is generally sent out clear, filtration being required to effect this.

·MISTURÆ VARIÆ.

SALTS IN MIXTURES.

SOME very soluble salts, such as acetate of potash or iodide of potassium, can be dissolved in the bottle with sufficient of the water prescribed. Those who object to keeping ready-made solutions have bottles of crystalline substances hand-powdered, so that they may be weighed out more quickly and dissolved more easily. When decoctions or infusions are ordered the salts can be readily dissolved in them while hot, but the dispenser must first assure himself if the quantity ordered is more than will remain dissolved in the cold solution, as in that case the salts will crystallise out. Carbonate of ammonia must be dissolved in cold water.

Nearly all salts dissolve to a greater extent in warm than in cold water. To this there are some notable exceptions—for example, some organic salts of the alkaline earths—but the exceptions are too insignificant to affect the rule. Sometimes the temperature makes an appreciable difference in the solubility of salts in a mixture. Thus, 100 parts of water will dissolve 35 to 40 parts of crystallised sulphate of soda in summer, while in cold winter nights water will not hold more than about 25 per cent. in solution.

In mixtures containing excess of powdered salts, such as chlorate of potash, the powder slowly assumes the form of large crystals. This is due to the mixture being exposed to variable temperatures, solution and crystallisation taking place alternately, the powder dissolving by preference. Little can be done to prevent the change, so that the dispenser should be ready with an explanation if complaint be made.

Many salts are more soluble if several are dissolved in the same vehicle, or if there is some acid present. Sulphate of potash, for instance, is more soluble in a solution of sulphate of magnesia than in pure water. In such cases double salts are formed, which are more soluble than the individual ones. In the case of 'Henry's Solution of Magnesia' the sulphuric acid makes the sulphate of magnesia dissolve in a smaller proportion of water than would otherwise be required.

The addition of tinctures, or other spirituous liquids, to a solution of a salt tends to throw the salt out of solution, because the mixture of spirit and water is not so good a solvent as water alone.

Liq. sodii arseniatis	ⅿ 96
Sp. vini rect.	ad ℨiij.

In this case much of the arseniate crystallises out in a few hours. When the prescription was received it was suggested to the doctor that the liquor should be mixed with ℥iss. of water and then ℥iss. of spirit added, as this solution yields no crystals. The alteration was immediately sanctioned.

MIXTURES CONTAINING INSOLUBLE OR SLIGHTLY SOLUBLE SUBSTANCES.

Such substances should always be rubbed down in a mortar with some of the fluid. If added to the mixture, many substances are liable to aggregate and float about in little balls, which are afterwards difficult to separate. Especially is this the case with vegetable powders, with carbonate of magnesia, calomel, and precipitated sulphur. Ipecacuanha should be added to the fluid and well shaken; if liquid be poured on it in an empty bottle it absorbs some and forms a doughy mass. The best plan is to rub it down with some syrup or mucilage, if any such is an ingredient of the mixture.

Benzoic Acid must be well powdered before mixing; it the prescription contains tinctures the acid should be dissolved in them, and the water added with a brisk shake.

Gallic Acid.—Cold water dissolves about 1 per cent.; hot water one-third of its weight ; it is freely soluble in glycerine and alcohol. To prepare glycerine solutions of gallic acid use a moderate heat, as high temperatures change it to pyrogallol and carbonic anhydride. When required in the form of ointment it should be dissolved with a few drops of alcohol before mixing with the fat.

Some vegetable ingredients require to be rubbed with sugar of milk before being made into mixtures. *All potent ingredients which are slow of solution, such as perchloride of mercury, strychnine, and the like, should be completely dissolved before they are placed in the bottle.*

EXTRACTS IN MIXTURES.

Solid extracts are seldom prescribed in mixture in this country, but they are on the Continent, and the following hints by Dr. Hager will be useful to the English dispenser.

When alcoholic extracts have to be dissolved in a mixture the vehicle in which they are rubbed down into solution should not be hot.

If purely resinous extracts have to be compounded in a mixture they should first be rubbed in a mortar with twice or three times their weight of powdered gum arabic, then combined with the vehicle perfectly cold. If any syrup is ordered in the mixture the resinous extract should be rubbed down with that. Example :—

Ammonii muriatici	5·0
Succi liquiritiæ	5·0
Aquæ destillatæ	100·0
Ext. cinæ æth.	1·5

M. et solve. D. S., &c.

The extract should be first rubbed with powdered gum arabic 1·5, and with the muriate of ammonia, then with the liquorice in concentrated solution, and, lastly, with the cold water.

Extracts made with water and alcohol are difficult to mix with a purely spirituous solution. Example :—

Extracti hyoscyami Ph. G.	•	•	•	•	1·0
Tincturæ valerianæ .	•	•	•	•	•	5·0
Spiritus ætherei	•	•	•	•	•	•	20·0

Misce.

In this prescription, the ethereal spirit being only an adjuvant, a slight modification must be made. The extract must be dissolved in 2 parts of distilled water, then the tincture of valerian, and 18 (instead of 20) parts of spirit of ether added. In the case where the fluid with which the extract is to be mixed is itself a strong medicine (tinct. digitalis æth., for example) nothing remains but to rub it with its own weight of water, and then rub the partial solution vigorously with the tincture.

Inspissated Juices are similarly treated; but, when dissolved in water, they should stand in a measure for two or three minutes to settle, and the fluid be poured off carefully from the sediment.

The narcotic non-resinous extracts can be kept in concentrated solutions. Ten parts of extract should be dissolved in a mixture of 12 parts of water, 4 parts of glycerine, and 4 parts of spirits of wine. When dispensing from these solutions three times the quantity of extract ordered must be weighed. The label should indicate this exactly. Some extracts, such as aconite, henbane, and belladonna, in solution, will require well shaking before weighing.

Lactucarium ought to be rubbed down in a mortar with twice its weight of sugar and a few drops of spirit of wine.

Refined Liquorice-juice can be kept in solution in its own weight of distilled water, or in a mixture of 3 parts of distilled water and 1 part of glycerine, in moderate-sized bottles quite full. Some acids and many salts of alkaloids can only be mixed with solution of liquorice in a very diluted condition, as they precipitate the glycyrrhizin and cause a very disagreeable appearance.

Extract of Opium forms peculiar flakes with the mucilage of carragheen, althæa, and salep, but it can be mixed with them if first rubbed down with syrup or dissolved in 50 times its weight of water. Acetate of lead is sometimes ordered in such a mixture, and this also should be dissolved in 50 times its weight of water before being added.

MISCELLANEOUS INGREDIENTS.

Acid. Carbolic.—A cold saturated solution in water contains 7 per cent. When a larger proportion is ordered in a mixture with water it can be suspended by triturating the acid with an equal quantity of mucilage of acacia, and gradually adding the water. This addition, however, should not be made without authority.

Acid. Hydrocyanic. Dil. is best measured with a long graduated syringe, and put into the bottle last. This will keep well if prepared as follows :—

Acid. hydrocyan. dil. B.P.	ℨj.
Glycerin.	ℨiij.
Aq.	ad ℥ij.

In corked bottles. Mixtures containing hydrocyanic acid should have a 'shake' label on. All strongly poisonous ingredients should be checked, if possible, by a second dispenser.

Acid. Salicylic.—Mention has already been made of the combination of quinine and salicylates. A similar change occurs in the following :—

Sodæ salicylat.	ℨiij.
Tinct. buchu	ℨvj.
Decoct. cinchon.	ad ℥viij.

Salicylate mixtures, as previously mentioned, are very apt to change colour. For example :—

Sodæ salicylat.	ℨij.
Ferri sulph.	Ɇj.
Pulv. tragac. co.	ℨj.
Syrup. aurantii	℥ss.
Aquæ chloroformi	ad ℥vj.

This forms a deep reddish mixture, due to the formation of salicylate of iron.

Salicylates are about the most delicate test for ferric salts, and, as it is impossible to preserve ferrous sulphate absolutely· from oxidation, it naturally follows that the mixture should be dark-coloured, whether it is prepared from salicylate made with natural or artificial acid. The sulphate of iron (granulated) should be dissolved in the syrup and 1 oz. of chloroform water; the salicylate and compound powder made into a mixture with the rest of the water, and the iron solution then added to it. In this way the most lightly coloured mixture is obtained.

Alkaloids.—A knowledge of the ordinary alkaloidal reactions is very useful at the dispensing-counter. The following is a fair example of the cases in which this knowledge may be turned to practical account. On the addition of liq. strychninæ, the mixture assumes a yellow colour :—

Liq. Donovan.	ℨij.
,, strychninæ	ℨj.
Syr. ferri iodidi	℥j.
Glycerini	ad ℥ij.

Strychnine and other alkaloids are precipitated by alkaline iodides, and especially by mercuric iodide (a solution of which in potassium iodide and water is known as Meyer's alkaloidal reagent). The precipitate in this case is an iodo-hydrargyrate of strychnine.

Ammonia and Bromides.—The following mixture becomes colourless after standing for a few days :—

Sodii bromidi	ʒiv.
Ammonii carbonatis	ʒj.
Tr. chlorof. co.	ℨij.
Aquæ	ad ℥viij.

The explanation of this appears to be that solutions of a halogen salt and free ammonia are very liable to undergo a change, with formation of a nitrogen bromide, etc. It is conceivable that if this were to take place the vegetable colouring matter would be destroyed during the process.

Bismuth Subnitrate and a Bicarbonate.—Subnitrate of bismuth reacts with bicarbonate of soda or potash with liberation of carbonic acid gas, the reaction being :—

$$2BiONO_3 + 2NaHCO_3 = Bi_2O_2CO_3 + 2NaNO_3 + H_2O + CO_2.$$

The reaction is sometimes slow, but if it does not occur in dispensing the prescription, it is apt to take place after the mixture is sent out. Some dispensers use subcarbonate of bismuth instead of the subnitrate, but this course cannot be followed without sanction. The best plan is to place the subnitrate and bicarbonate in a mortar and pour a little boiling water upon them, when effervescence takes place immediately.

Cocaine and Carbolic Acid.—The following prescription illustrates the importance of using only distilled water for dispensing purposes :—

Cocain. hydroch.	gr. x.
Glycer. carbol.	ʒij.
Aquæ	ad ℥ij.

The method followed by the correspondent who received this prescription was to dissolve the cocaine hydrochlorate in 1 oz. of water; the glycerine in 1 oz. ; the latter added in portions to the former. The first portion caused no precipitation, the subsequent portions increasing precipitates.

On putting the matter to test we obtained a perfectly clear mixture with distilled water, but spring water gave a milky mixture, due evidently to the precipitation of cocaine hydrate, owing to the carbonate of lime in the water. Carbolic acid gives a milky mixture with solution of cocaine hydrochlorate in distilled water, but no apparent precipitate.

Ether should never be mixed with hot fluids. This applies equally to all volatile substances, such, for example, as hydrocyanic acid, and, as a rule, when they require to be added to any mixture not of the nature of an emulsion, they should invariably be added last in order. Imagine the result of pouring a drachm of strong liquor ammonia into an empty 8-oz. bottle, then filling with some other fluid ; the chances are that at least one-fourth of the ammonia will be dissipated.

To dissolve volatile oils in water it is best to warm the water up to about 100° F. and filter out so much of the oil as remains undissolved, unless sugar be ordered in the mixture, when the oil is rubbed down therewith, making an oleo-saccharate, or, if spirit or ether be ordered, the oil is dissolved therein.

Liquor Bismuthi et Ammon. Cit.—We have already referred to the difference between the old liquor and the new. The following is another example :—.

Liq. bismuth.	℥ij.
Liq. magnes. bicarb.	℥iss.
Aq. chlorof.	ad ℥vj.

A chemist dispensed this mixture clear, and it was returned as being different from that previously dispensed, which had a thick white deposit. He procured two samples of liq. bismuthi from local firms : result, in both cases, a mixture slightly milky. Next Schacht's liq. bismuthi was tried : result, a clear mixture.

We compounded the prescription with the B.P. 1885 solution, freshly prepared, the result being a mixture containing a copious white deposit of bismuth carbonate. This result cannot be avoided. With the old liquor a clear mixture was obtained. The new liq. bismuth. et ammon. citrat. is a very different preparation from the old liquor, and from its proto-type, liquor bismuthi (Schacht). The old liquor contained a large excess of citrate of ammonia, and this excess prevents the precipitation of bismuth.

Tinct. ferri perchlor.	℥iij.
Liq. bismuthi	℥iss.
Acid. phosph. conc. B.P.	℥ij.
Tr. nucis vom.	℥iij.
Tr. quassiæ	℥iv.
Bromid. potass.	℥iv.

This can be made into a clear mixture by first mixing the tinct. ferri perchlor. with the phosphoric acid in a glass measure, then adding the two tinctures; afterwards gradually adding the liq. bismuthi, constantly stirring with a glass rod, and lastly adding the potassium bromide in fine powder.

Liquor Pepticus.—A correspondent asked us if the following mixture should be dispensed with or without a sediment :—

Liq. peptici (Benger's)	ʒiij.
Sodæ bicarb.	ʒiv.
.Glycerini.	ʒvj.
Inf. quassiæ	ad ʒviij.

To this Mr. Baden Benger replied: 'I find the prescription yields a clear mixture, which, after standing several days, shows no sign of sediment. *Liquor Pepticus* (Benger) is slightly acid, and will cause effervescence when mixed with *Sodæ bicarb.* It is difficult to see the object of the prescriber in this case, as pepsin and its preparations are practically inert in any but acid media. This mixture is strongly alkaline, and the pepsin would certainly have to wait its turn, till after the soda had been neutralised by the acid contents of the stomach.'

Pulv. Tragacanth.—In a mixture with tincture, put the tincture into the bottle, shake so as to cover the sides, then add the tragacanth, and shake. If no tincture is ordered, put about ʒss. or ʒj. of spirit into a measure, add the tragacanth, and stir up with a glass rod, then add the water, etc., or do the same thing in the bottle, which must be dry. The following is a Bloomsbury Square examination prescription :—

Bismuthi subnit.	ʒj.
Sodii bicarb.	ʒj.
Pulv. tragacanth	ʒss.
Syrup simpl.	ʒiij.
Tr. cardam. co.	ʒij.
Aq. dest.	ad ʒvj.

Fiat mist. One-sixth part t.d.s.

The reaction between the soda and bismuth has already been noted. As regards the tragacanth, a dispenser would not hesitate in the pharmacy to take an equivalent quantity of the mucilage, but the candidate may not adopt this procedure in the examination-room. Two methods may occur to him: (1) to mix the powders in a mortar and add the water (hot in order to force the chemical action) gradually; or (2) to treat the tragacanth in a dry state with the tincture, in a similar way to the official process for making the mucilage. A combination of the two methods is best.

Tinctura Hyoscyami made with ·biennial leaves, when mixed with water, should present a decidedly cloudy appearance. Tincture made with the annual leaves also gives a cloudy mixture, but not so much so as in the case of the biennial.

Vinum Ferri and Alkalies.—

Vin. ferri B.P. .	℥iv.
Potass. bicarb. .	ℨijss.
Tr. nucis vom. .	♏lxxx.

If the wine of iron is properly made, it gives a precipitate of carbonate of iron with the potash. Some houses send out a mixture like this clear. A case of this kind was thoroughly investigated, and it was found that the wine of iron which had been used to make a clear mixture contained only a trace of iron, and what there was in it was kept in solution owing to the presence of citrate of potash. Vinum ferri and liquor arsenicalis are sometimes prescribed together, the result being a repulsive-looking muddy mixture; liquor arsenici hydrochlor. should be used instead of the alkaline solution.

MIXTURES WITH RESINOUS TINCTURES.

Resinous tinctures (ginger, nux vomica, hops, etc.), when dispensed in aqueous solutions, should have a 'shake the bottle' label attached, especially when acids are present; so also should infusions of cinchona or cascarilla, decoction of aloes, cinchona, or sarsaparilla, or any preparations *likely* to give a deposit on standing a few days. A patient seeing a sediment is always doubtful whether it should be taken or not, and a 'shake' never does harm, even if no precipitate occurs.

Tinctures of guaiacum and Indian hemp cannot be dispensed in aqueous mixtures unless mucilage or a similar substance is used. The best *modus operandi* is to take a measure of acacia mucilage equal to that of the tincture, dilute it with three measures of water, pour in the tincture, gently agitate, and dilute further if necessary. If much water has to be added, the finished mixture should not contain less than ♏xx. or ℨss. of mucilage to the ounce. With skilful manipulation many resinous mixtures (*e.g.* guaiacum, myrrh, sumbul, etc.) can be diffused through water so as to produce a presentable mixture without the aid of mucilage; but if such be violently agitated the resin soon separates in lumps, and, even if allowed to remain undisturbed, it will subside and adhere tenaciously to the sides of the bottle; consequently, if the resin be of a potent nature the use of mucilage or similar agent is imperative. Syrups, even if present in considerable quantity, do not effectually prevent deposition of the resin. The following is a fair example of the kind of mixtures referred to :—

Vin. colchici	ℨj.
Potass. bicarb.	ℨss.
Tinct. cannab. ind.	ℨss.
Spt. ammon. co.	ℨj.
Tinct. calumbœ	ℨij.
Tinct. gentianœ	ℨij.
Aquœ	ad ℥vj.

A good mixture may be made as follows: Mix in a dry measure the tincture of cannabis with the sal volatile and other tinctures, and dissolve the potash in about 4 oz. of water, and add the wine. Now make a small cone of white demy with a small opening at the apex. Immerse the apex of the cone just beneath the surface of the bicarbonate solution (which may be held in a 4-oz. measure), and shoot in the tinctures through the cone, which must be quickly more deeply immersed at the same time, and a little suggestive manipulation will turn out a mixture in every respect satisfactory. A slight precipitation only will take place after several hours' standing.

When we come to deal with large quantities of resinous tinctures we require the addition of mucilage :—

Potassii iodidi	℥iss.
Tr. cimicifug.	℥j.
Tr. guaiaci am.	℥j.
Tr. nucis vom.	℥iss.
Aq. chloroformi.	ad ℥iv.

A good mixture can only be obtained by the addition of acacia. Make a mucilage of 2 drachms of the powdered gum with $\frac{1}{2}$ oz. of chloroform water ; dissolve the iodide in the rest of the water, and mix the mucilage with it ; then mix the tincture of guaiacum with the other tinctures and add to the whole of the watery mixture with brisk agitation.

Some extracts form a good substitute for mucilage, thus :—

Tinct. cannabis indic.	℥iv.
Tinct. digitalis	℥j.
Ext. taraxaci	℥iv.
Ammon. chlor.	℥iv.
Aq. chlorof.	ad ℥vj.

Rub the extract down with about 2 oz. of the water, pour in the mixed tinctures, nearly fill the bottle with aq. chlorof., and add the ammon. chlor.

Sp. æth. nit.	℥ss.
Tinct. tolut.	℥ss.
Tinct. camph. co.	℥j.

If this be mixed in different ways it will present different appearances. The principle to be borne in mind here, as in all similar cases, is that it is far easier to keep a substance in solution than it is to take it up again after precipitation. In the instance before us it is evident that the substances should be mixed in the order of their percentage of alcohol—that is, the spirit of nitre should be mixed with the tolu, and the tinct. camph. co. added last, and by degrees, with agitation. This pre-scription furnishes another example of the necessity of attending fully to the instructions of the Pharmacopœia, if uniformity in dispensing is to be arrived at. It would not matter how skilfully the chemist manipulated, if his tinct. camph. co. were

made with 'proof spirit'—not yet extinct in chemists' shops—
made by mixing equal parts of rectified spirit and water; he
could not get the bright transparent mixture which is afforded
when the official tincture is used.

In the following prescription for a 'vapour' we have a
troublesome difficulty to get over—viz. to keep the benzoin
and other resinous ingredients from forming a magma :—

Thymol hydrat.	gr. xxx.
Spt. chloroform.	ʒiij.
Tinct. benzoin co.	ʒiij.
Magnes. calc. levis	gr. x.
Aquæ	ad ℥ij.

The best plan in this case is to mix the tincture and the
spirit, and dissolve the thymol in the mixture. Then mix the
magnesia with 10 drachms of water, and pour the spirituous
mixture into it. Light magnesia must be used.

Here it may be remarked that the light carbonate of
magnesia is largely employed in making the quasi-emulsion
inhalations of such essential oils as Oleum Pini Sylvestris,
Oleum Pini Pumilionis (Pumiline), etc. These are generally
dispensed by mixing with a small quantity of the light carbonate in a mortar and adding the water. In this way the use
of spirit, which might be therapeutically inapplicable in some
throat cases, is avoided.

If, notwithstanding all precautions, the resin separates in
unpleasant-looking particles, these must be collected on a previously damped strainer and rubbed down in a mortar with a
little powdered gum arabic and a few drops of water. One
mixture of an alcoholic solution of a resin with water may be
mentioned as a useful cosmetic, making, it has frequently been
stated, a perfectly suspended milky compound. It is known
as *Lait Virginal*, and is composed of—

Tinct. benzoini	ʒij.
Aquæ rosæ	℥vj.

Try how you will, you cannot succeed in making an in-
separable mixture without the addition of a few drachms of
mucilage of acacia.

EMULSIONS.

THIS class of preparations gives as much trouble to the dispenser as anything that comes to the dispensing-counter.

Emulsions are made in several ways—as, for example, by making a soap, as when an alkali is added to a fixed oil ; by suspending a resinous substance in a mucilaginous liquid, as in copaiba emulsion, or in mistura ammoniaci and mistura guaiaci of the Pharmacopœia. By yolk of egg, as with turpentine, or castor-oil.

An emulsion is perfect when the oil-globules are invisible to the naked eye. Something short of this may look well and give very fair results, but it is only when the more perfect form is attained that it can safely and properly fulfil all its requirements in dispensing. Emulsions made with tragacanth, such as cod-liver-oil emulsion, may show globules of oil and yet not separate. This is the case with the following from the *Physicians' Pharmacopœia*, which was for a time semi-officialized in the British Pharmaceutical Conference formulary :—

Pure cod-liver-oil	. 40 oz.
Powd. tragacanth	. 200 gr.
Tinct. benzoin (1 oz. to 10 oz. S.V.R.)	. $\frac{1}{2}$ oz.
Spirit chloroform	. $\frac{1}{3}$,,
Glycerine	. 2 ,,
Ess. of almonds	. 40 mins.
,, oil lemon	. 40 ,,
Distilled water	to 80 oz.
Calcium hypophos.	. 10 dr. 40 gr.
Sodium ,, ...	. 2 ,, 40 ,,
Potassium ,, ...	. 1 ,, 20 ,,

M

Place the oil in a Winchester quart, and pour into it the powdered tragacanth, tincture of benzoin, and spirit of chloroform mixed; agitate briskly for one minute, then add all at once a pint of distilled water and agitate as before; lastly, add the oils, glycerine, and remaining water, with hypo-phosphites dissolved in it. This emulsion is said to keep good for years.

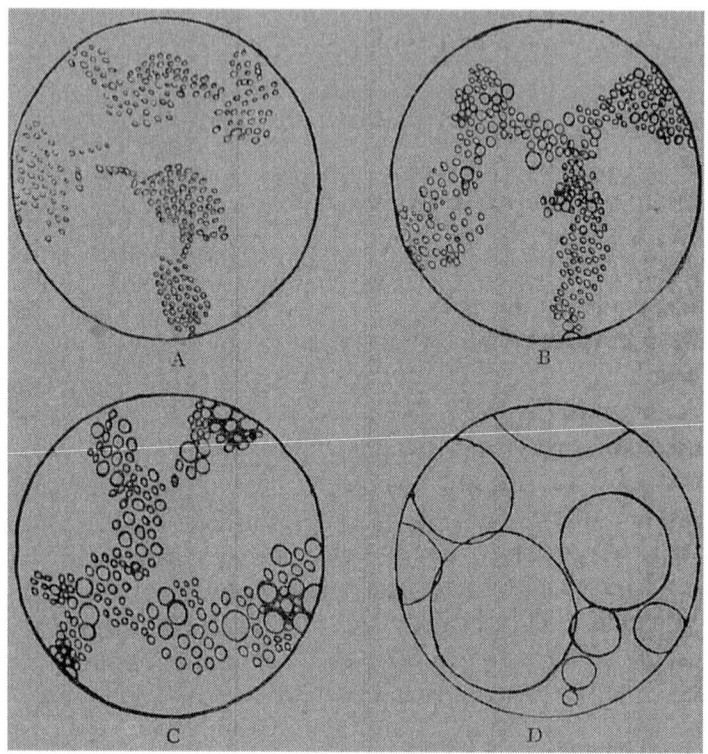

The above figures illustrate the various degrees of perfection and badness shown by emulsions. A shows the appearance of milk under the microscope; B is a cod-liver-oil emulsion made with the yolk of egg; C cod-liver-oil emulsion made with acacia; and D made with tragacanth, according to the *Physician's Pharmacopœia.* These are magnified about 100 diameters.

The readiest method of producing an emulsion of oils is to triturate 1 part of powdered gum arabic in a mortar with 2 parts of oil, add at one time $1\frac{1}{2}$ part of water, and triturate, when, after a few turns of the pestle, the whole is emulsified. The rest of the water may be added by degrees. At least 3 parts of powdered gum are required for 8 parts of an essential oil, and 2 parts for 8 parts of fixed oils and balsams, but double these quantities are generally required, according to the amount of water which is present.

If we shake up a fixed oil with water, we break it up into a multitude of minute particles, so that the entire mixture has a milky appearance, but if allowed to stand the oil speedily separates. This is owing to two causes—the lesser specific gravity of the oil and the want of adhesion between its particles and those of the water. The art of making emulsions consists in finding and introducing some body to overcome this antagonism, so that when at rest the mixture shall not separate. The emulsifying media vary as stated, but the principle of action is the same in every case. The object is to break up the substance to be emulsified into minute particles, and to enclose each of them in a coating of the emulsifying agent. The following examples are instructive :—

Bals. copaib.	ʒvj.
Pulv. acaciæ	ʒiij.
Sp. æth. nit.	ʒij.
Aquæ	ad ℥vj.

Make a thick mucilage with the gum and a little water, then add with constant trituration, alternately, first a little of the oleo-resin, then a little water, and so on till the whole of the copaiba is emulsified ; place in a bottle, add more water, and, lastly, the sp. æth. nit. By such procedure the copaiba is minutely divided, and each particle coated with mucilage. If the mucilage were added to the copaiba, or even the whole of the copaiba added at once to the mucilage, a different result would be effected. The copaiba would doubtless be broken up, but instead of being coated by, it would form the covering of, particles of mucilage, and on standing would quickly separate.

Ol. amygdal. dulc.	ʒiv.
Liq. potassæ	ʒj.
Vin. ipecac.	ʒj.
Aquæ	ad ℥iv.

Mix the liq. potassæ with 3 drachms of water, add the oil, shake until thoroughly emulsified, add more water, and the vin. ipecac. last.

Our next example is an examination prescription upon which a candidate failed:—

Ol. ricini	.	.	.	.	.	.	℥iss.
Mucil. acac.	.	.	.	.	.	.	ℨj.
Syrup.	.	.	.	.	.	.	ℨss.
Tr. zingib.	.	.	.	.	.	.	♏ xv.
Aq.	.	.	.	.	.	.	ad ℥iss.

Rub the oil down with 28 grains of pulv. acacia (which is the equivalent of ℨj. of mucilage), and when that is thoroughly mixed add all at once ℨj. of water, after which triturate until the whole is emulsified ; gradually add more water in small quantities ; lastly add the syrup and tinct. zingib., both previously diluted with a little water. Made according to these directions a uniform preparation is produced which does not separate until kept for some time. The prescription is not a difficult one, but requires careful manipulation. In making emulsions it should be borne in mind that syrups, and preparations containing spirit, should invariably be added last.

The question as to whether emulsions of oils and oleo-resins should be made with mortar and pestle or in a bottle has been often discussed, and need not be entered on here, it now being almost universally agreed that the mortar and pestle are best, and a broad pestle should always be used.

EMULSIFICATION OF SPECIAL DRUGS.

Balsam of Peru may be emulsified with yolk of egg or with powdered acacia, as in the following:—

Potass. acet.	.	.	.	.	.	.	℥ss.
Acid. salicylic.	.	.	.	.	.	.	ℨj.
Liq. morph. acet.	.	.	.	.	.	.	ℨij.
Balsam. peru.	.	.	.	.	.	.	℥ss.
Aquæ	.	.	.	.	.	.	ad ℥viij.

Rub up the balsam with 4 drachms of powdered acacia, exactly as was done in the case of the last example, using from 5 to 6 oz. of water for dilution. Separately rub together the acid and acetate with the morphia solution and the rest of the water. Mix the two.

Balsam of Tolu.—

Dissolve—

	Parts
Balsam of tolu	2
Alcohol 90°	10
Tincture of quillaia	10
Water	78

(See special remarks regarding the use of tincture of quillaia.)

Benzoin (tinctura).—The simple tincture makes a good emulsion with a little mucilage, and the compound tincture may be emulsified with yolk of egg or mucilage, the yolk of egg giving a more stable emulsion.

Copaiba Resin.—Rub the resin with one-third its weight of sugar of milk, and about its own weight of pulv. acaciæ, and add the water gradually. Mr. Gerrard recommends the resin to be rubbed with twice its weight of compound powder of almonds until well incorporated, adding the water after the manner of forming an emulsion.

Chloroform is made into an excellent emulsion by using $\frac{1}{2}$ drachm of the tincture of quillaia to every 10 minims of chloroform.

Oleum Cadini (Juniper Tar Oil) may, according to the Société de Pharmacie de Paris, be made into emulsions in the same way as balsam of tolu. Various methods are given throughout this chapter.

Spermaceti may be emulsified with yolk of egg after being very finely powdered with rectified spirit.

Terebene may be emulsified in the same way as turpentine. The following recipe is a fairly difficult one to compound :—

Terebene	3j.
Sp. chloroform.	3ij.
Tinct. tolu	3ij.
Syr. tolu	3vj.
Aq. menth. pip.	ad 3vj.

Make a mucilage with 4 drachms of acacia and 6 drachms of peppermint-water in a mortar; of this reserve 2 drachms;

with the remainder in the mortar rub the terebene until emulsified, and dilute with 2 ounces of peppermint-water. Dilute the reserved 2 drachms of mucilage with peppermint-water; transfer to a bottle, and with this emulsify the tincture of tolu; to this add the terebene emulsion and finally the other ingredients.

Another method of making the emulsion is the following: Pour 1 ounce of mucilage into the bottle, add the tolu and terebene, shake thoroughly, then add the other ingredients. A beautiful emulsion is formed. The tolu appears to accelerate the process, probably owing to the fact of its being more easily assimilated.

Tinctura Guaiaci Ammoniata.—When ordered in an aqueous mixture, take the same quantity of mucilage as tincture; dilute with twice as much water; pour into the bottle and shake to wet the whole inner surface. The tincture should then be added and shaken vigorously, and the rest of the water added gradually.

Turpentine.—Yolk of egg emulsifies turpentine well. Triturate the yolk carefully in a mortar, add gradually twice its volume of water, and strain through muslin. Of this mixture transfer to a bottle a measure equal to, or slightly more than, the turpentine to be emulsified, shake, add the whole of the turpentine, shake until thoroughly emulsified, and dilute further if necessary. It may also be satisfactorily emulsified with acacia (powder or mucilage).

Terebinthina Chia.—This substance was vaunted as a cure for cancer some years ago, and its introducer, Dr. Clay, of Birmingham, still retains faith in it; and for that reason the drug is still prescribed occasionally, generally in the form of an emulsion of the ethereal solution of turpentine with tragacanth and sulphur. The latter is an essential ingredient; indeed, Mr. Valentine Knaggs says it is the sulphur, and not the turpentine, which does the good. The emulsion is made by mixing ½ an ounce of the solution of turpentine (1 ounce in 2 of absolute ether) with 40 grains of sulphur, and 24 grains of tragacanth;

add 6 ounces of water, stirring briskly, then an ounce of syrup and water to 16 ounces. The addition of an ounce of acacia mucilage makes a better emulsion.

RECENT METHODS.

Casein.—We owe the idea of making emulsions with casein to M. Léger, a Parisian pharmacist, who communicated a paper on the subject to the Paris Pharmaceutical Society in April 1887. The following are the principal points of his communication : Natural emulsions are made with bodies of an albuminous character. In milk, the model of emulsions, butter is kept in suspension by casein. Then why not try to separate out the butter and obtain the casein of the milk in a soluble condition, and then see what sort of emulsion will result? The first step, the elimination of the fatty substance, is best performed by means of ammonia. The separation is not so perfect as when such a solvent as ether is employed ; but it is sufficient for practical purposes, and more convenient with large quantities of liquid. Take 4 litres of milk and 60 grammes of ammonia (say 1 gallon of milk and $2\frac{1}{2}$ oz. solution of ammonia), and after shaking well set the liquor aside for twenty-four hours. Two layers are now observed, the semi-saponified butter above and the lacto-serum below. The lower liquid is drawn off, and casein is precipitated from it by acetic acid. The magma is collected and strongly pressed, to expel moisture ; now add by trituration 10 grammes of bicarbonate of soda, and, finally, mix in enough sugar to obtain a powder representing when dry about 10 per cent. of its weight of casein. The preparation keeps well in securely corked bottles for at least three years. It has a slight, not unpleasant, smell, which is not appreciable in preparations.

Now as to the way to use it. M. Léger divides substances to be emulsified into two classes—that is, (1) those soluble in alcohol, and (2) those insoluble. The first class, which includes resins, balsams, oleo-resins, etc., can be worked very simply in the bottle itself. The product is first weighed or measured into the bottle, and enough alcohol is added to dissolve it. Then for a 4-oz. mixture about 10 grammes (2½ drachms) of saccharated casein, dissolved in an equal weight of water, is added and thoroughly shaken, after which the remaining water, etc., are gradually introduced, with continual shaking. With class (2)—that is, ordinary oils—a mortar is needed. The manipulation is the same as when gum arabic is used.

The emulsions thus formed are more perfect and more stable than those obtained with any other emulsive agent. But their greatest merit, M. Léger claims, is that they are more palatable, and more easily supported by the stomach. Castor-oil, for instance, which to children has to be administered in the liquid state, since they cannot take capsules, he found to be readily accepted and retained by the most delicate stomachs. The same patients could not retain the oil emulsified with gum arabic or tragacanth.

SUBSTITUTES FOR GUM ACACIA.

Irish Moss.—Cod-liver-oil emulsions have long been prepared with Irish moss, but the emulsifying properties of the moss do not appear to have been systematically studied.

Recently Mr. Peter Boa (Edinburgh) gave his attention to the matter, and made various proposals. First, as to the difficulty of obtaining a clear mucilage, he stated that he found that by using a hot-water funnel and straining the mucilage through absorbent cotton-wool supported on muslin a preparation clear enough for all but exceptional purposes could be obtained with comparatively little difficulty. If a perfectly water-clear preparation be required, it may be obtained by making a weak mucilage, filtering it clear, and then evaporating to the required consistency. The mucilage is prepared by digesting ¼ oz. of washed moss in 24 oz. of water for an hour. boiling for five minutes, and straining the moss mucilage. It serves as well as acacia for chalk mixture ; guaiacum mixture prepared with it has not so green a colour as that made with acacia. For suspending copaiba it is superior to acacia—separation takes place much more slowly and less completely. Part of the copaiba remains in an emulsified state at the bottom of the bottle when moss is used, but with acacia the whole rises to the top. For emulsifying cod-liver-oil it is greatly superior to acacia for preventing separation, but finer division of the oil is obtained with acacia. Moss mucilage ʒvj., cod-liver-oil ʒj., and water ʒij. produce an emulsion that does not readily separate. Using ʒvj. acacia mucilage, ʒj. cod-liver-oil, and ʒij. water, the resulting emulsion soon. separates. It is *not* adapted for suspending heavy powders, such as bismuth sub-nitrate. The mucilage keeps well in full bottles. Mr. Emlen Painter has suggested that the moss mucilage should be eva-porated and scaled, and the scales dissolved when required for making an emulsion.

Gelatine has also been proposed as an emulsifying agent, especially for paraffin oils, and is the subject of a patent (No. 3,466. 1886). According to this patent a solution of gelatine or other similar substance is made, in the proportion of 4 oz. to the gallon of water. In 12 parts of this 1 part of phosphate of soda or potash, or carbonate of soda or potash, is dissolved by the aid of heat, and this mixture is capable, by the ordinary means, of emulsifying from 24 to 36 parts of animal or vege-table oils. For embrocations ammonia is substituted for the above-named salts. Chloroform and such liquids may be emulsified in this manner. For mineral oils and the like the alkali is replaced by soft soap. For example, an emulsify-ing solution is made with 6 oz. of concentrated size, 1 lb. of soft soap, and 1 gallon of water, and this mixture is capable of emulsifying 2 gallons of paraffin oil. The method is only likely to be useful in veterinary dispensing.

Senega Root and Quillaia Bark contain a principle (saponin) which possesses powerful emulsifying properties, and imparts to infusions of either of these drugs the frothing property which is not the least important of their characteristics. Mr. H. Collier, teacher of pharmacy at Guy's Hospital, studied the use of a tincture of quillaia in the preparation of emulsions, and presented his results in the form of a paper to the British Pharmaceutical Conference. From this we take the following hints:—The tincture is made by digesting 4 oz. of the coarsely powdered inner bark in 1 pint of rectified spirit for a week, then filtering. If a little of this tincture is shaken up with mercury the metal is quickly divided into fine particles, and is prevented from reuniting. The tincture is peculiarly valuable for converting an oil into an emulsion in presence of an acid ; for example :—

Cod-liver-oil	℥j.
Glycerine	℥j.
Lime-juice	℥j.
Tincture of quillaia	ℨij.

This forms a very good emulsion. *Ext. filicis maris* is a troublesome substance to emulsify; milk being one of the best vehicles. Although it may with care be turned into a perfect emulsion with acacia, the mixture is not at all pleasing in character. The following is, however, all that can be desired :—

Ext. filicis maris	ℨj.
Tinct. quillaiæ	ℨss.
Aq. destill.	ad ℥j.
Misce.	

Oil of turpentine works well with its own measure of the tincture—*e.g.* :—

Ol. terebinthinæ	♏ xx.
Tinct. quillaiæ	♏ xx.
Aq. destillatæ	ad ℥j.
Misce.	

Resinous tinctures require more than their own volume of the quillaia tincture to prevent separation of resin ; thus :—

Tinct. tolutan.	♏ xl.
Tinct. quillaiæ	ℨj.
Aq. destillat.	ad ℥j.
Misce.	

After a short time the resin deposits, but it readily diffuses on shaking. It will be found that in cases of this kind acacia acts better—it gives viscosity to the liquid, and thus helps to retain the separated resin. For the same reason acacia or tragacanth is better for resin of copaiba than quillaia—in fact, quillaia is at its best with oils and oleo-resins, and should be avoided for resins.

HAGER ON EMULSIONS.

IN the original treatise considerable space was occupied by extracts from Dr. Hager on this subject. Emulsions are much more employed on the Continent than in this country, and the methods there pursued can be relied upon generally. We here reproduce the more important of Dr. Hager's hints, with editorial comments. This chapter will be found very useful to those who have German prescriptions to dispense.

Emulsions are, according to Dr. Hager, milky-looking, thick fluids, of mucilaginous or gummy substances, or combinations of water with oily, fatty, or resinous bodies. They are classified as seed, oil, balsam, gum-resin, resin, wax, or spermaceti emulsions.

SEED EMULSIONS

are made from seeds containing a fixed oil, such as almonds, poppy or hemp-seeds, etc., by crushing these and rubbing them with water. If necessary, the seeds are first washed several times with water; when clean, they are beaten, with about one-tenth their weight of water, into a soft mass, which, when taken between the fingers, reveals no albuminous lumps. The remainder of the fluid is then added gradually, with continual rubbing, until the whole is evenly suspended. The emulsion should lastly be strained through a clean coarse cloth (millers' cloth).

The small proportion ot oil contained in the seeds is suspended in the water by means of the albumen and mucilage of the seeds, but, if the latter are first rubbed down dry, the oil is expressed, and, though it is taken up in the emulsion, it more quickly separates, generally as a cream.

Almonds are always decorticated before being made into an emulsion, unless an order to the contrary is expressed.

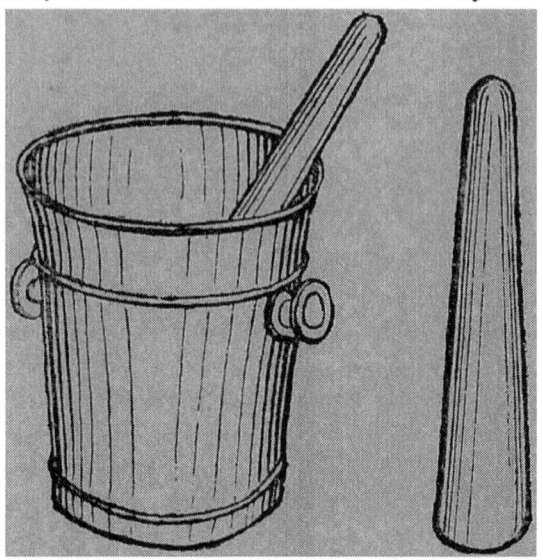

Poppy-seeds should be softened before being beaten, by letting them rest for five to ten minutes in warm—not hot—water.

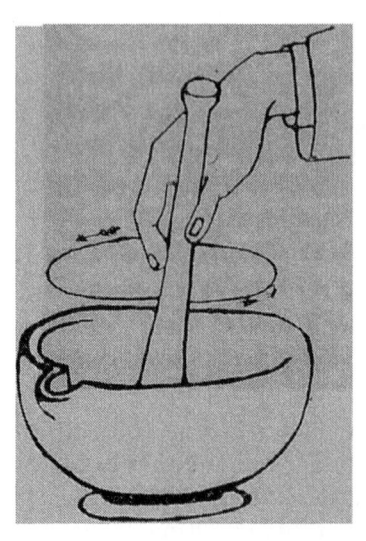

Highly polished brass mortars and marble mortars have been used for making emulsions, but within the last twenty years mortars have been made of a special kind of very hard porcelain, particularly for emulsions. The pestle is made of boxwood, and the forms of both pestle and mortar are shown in the above engraving. The height varies from five to eight inches. The boxwood pestle allows a good force to be used in crushing seeds without danger of injury to the porcelain. [An ordinary wedgewood mortar and pestle should be used for oil emulsions.

The second figure on page 172 shows such a mortar and the way in which the pestle should be used.—ED.]

Seed emulsions must not be made very hot, nor must hot fluids be added to them, or the albumen will be coagulated.

Lycopodium—a seed-like substance containing oil—may be made into an emulsion. After sifting to free it from coarse impurities, it is rubbed in a mortar with a little water until a damp crumbly mass is obtained. An addition of gum arabic is desirable to get a good emulsion. Then syrup or water is added gradually. If gum arabic be added, the prescription should be marked stating the quantity, 'Emulgendo admixtum.'

An oil, such as castor-oil, is sometimes ordered with a seed emulsion, as in the following :—

	Grammes
Amygdal. dulc.	20
Olei ricini	30
Aq. fœniculi	100
,, destill.	100
Sodæ nitrat.	15
Syrupi sacchari	25

M. F. emulsio

This is really a double emulsion.

OIL AND BALSAM EMULSIONS.

Fixed oils, such as almond, poppy, olive, linseed, and castor ; and balsams, such as copaiba and Peru, are easily combined with water by means of emulsifiers, of which gum arabic is the best. Yolk of egg and tragacanth are also emulsifiers. An emulsion with oil cannot be made satisfactorily with less gum arabic than one-fourth the weight of the oil. The proportion of water should be at least half of the total weight of the oil and gum.

The emulsifying power of 10 parts of gum arabic is estimated as equal to the yolk of a large hen's egg, to 1·25 part tragacanth, 1 part of salep.

These emulsions may be made in either of three ways

(1) By adding the water to the powdered gum in a large mixture mortar, mixing with a large-knobbed pestle ; then adding the oil or balsam all at once, and stirring till emulsified, which will require two or three minutes. This is generally the surest plan. .[With this remark we cannot agree.—ED.] Or (2) the gum may be put in the mortar, the oil poured on the top of it, the water round it, and then all the substances quickly stirred together. This is the method mostly adopted. Or (3) the oil may be rubbed with the gum, and the water added gradually. The proportions for a good emulsion are :—

	Parts
Oil or balsam	10
Gum arabic	5
Water to make the emulsion	7·5
,, add to the emulsion	77·5

The first method of emulsification described is not quite so speedy, but it is very sure. Sometimes castor-oil or balsam of copaiba cannot be emulsified by the second or third process. Probably this happens in consequence of some peculiarity in the oil or balsam, and the fact that in the two latter cases the gum is not dissolved quickly enough to affect the emulsification.

[The third plan is the plan which is now followed in this country and recommended by our leading pharmacists. Expertness is, however, required in order to have successful results. The probability is that moderately good results may be obtained by any one of the processes IF THE DISPENSER IS IN THE HABIT OF FOLLOWING IT. If he gets good results from any particular process we would not advise any experiments in the way of changing it. An emulsion at the best is a ticklish affair, and we have generally found it better to let well alone.—ED.]

Salts, extracts, or other solid bodies to be dissolved in emulsions should be separately dissolved in some of the water to be added, and mixed with the emulsion. If mixed with the emulsifier a separation of some of the oil will occur.

Lycopodium, which is often ordered with oil emulsions, causes such a separation with remarkable rapidity. It is best to emulsify the oil and the lycopodium separately, and to mix the two in diluted form.

Borax added to a gum-arabic emulsion converts the latter into a jelly. Diluted acetic acid restores the fluidity, but such an addition is by no means justifiable. If an emulsion with borax and gum be ordered in a prescription, the mixture must be sent out in a wide-mouthed bottle. The gelatinisation will not result till several hours after the mixing.

Balsam of Peru to be combined with an oil emulsion should be mixed with two-thirds of its weight of water, and stirred in with the emulsion in a mortar.

[The better plan is to mix about $\frac{1}{2}$ part stronger alcohol with 1 part glycerine, and to this add the balsam of Peru, and incorporate thoroughly. This may be diluted to a proper miscible point for an emulsion by the further addition of water, plain, or, better still, a mixture of glycerine and water gradually added.—Ed.]

Emulsions with tragacanth do not keep well, and are but seldom ordered. For their preparation 1 gramme of tragacanth is mixed with 20 grammes of water. To this 20 grammes of oil and 10 grammes of water are added at once, and combined into an emulsion with constant stirring. The rest of the water is added gradually.

[This is a mistake, as the many preparations now sold under the name of cod-liver-oil emulsion prepared with tragacanth sufficiently testify. It presents properties as an emulsifying agent which in many respects are unequalled for such an oil as cod-liver.—Ed.]

If spirits of wine, concentrated acids, solutions of salts, or tannin substances are to be mixed with emulsions, they should always be added in as diluted a form as possible.

Emulsions of Gum Resins.—The gum resins, such as galbanum, ammoniacum, myrrh, asafœtida, scammony, contain gummy matter, as well as resin insoluble in water, so that the addition of an emulsifier is not absolutely required. It is generally only necessary to rub down the gum resin to as fine a powder as possible, and emulsify with water. In warm weather this is not always practicable, as the gum resin is too soft. It is then best to put it into a mixture mortar in small pieces, sprinkle it with water, and put the mortar with the pestle in a moderately warm place until the substance has become of the consistence of honey. To each gramme of the gum resin are added 1 drop of almond-oil and 3 drops of mucilage of acacia, and then, by the gradual addition of warm water and vigorous working with the pestle, a good emulsion will be obtained.

Generally gum arabic or yolk of egg is ordered with a gum resin to emulsify it better. If either of these is used the gum resin should be in very fine powder. One part of gum arabic to 2 parts of gum resin or one yolk of egg to 20 grammes of gum resin is the usual proportion. If the gum resin cannot be powdered it is softened by warming, as explained, but with yolk of egg the temperature must not exceed 60° C.

Emulsions of Resins.—These are prepared from Venice turpentine, guaiacum resin, resin of jalap, and such-like substances.

Venice turpentine is easily emulsified by its own weight of gum arabic or by yolk of egg (two yolks to 20 grammes).

Resin of guaiacum is finely powdered and rubbed in a mortar with half its weight of gum arabic, water being added gradually. This emulsion assumes a bluish tint, varying in intensity according to the degree of concentration. The blue gradually changes to a green. A few drops of sweet spirit of nitre will develop the blue tint, as will also exposure to the air.

Resin of jalap is sometimes combined with almonds into an emulsion (two blanched sweet almonds to $\frac{1}{2}$ gramme of resin); but it soon separates. If neither almonds nor egg be ordered, but only gum or sugar, it is generally best to rub the resin first with its own weight of spirit before mixing with water.

Quinoidine and some other amorphous alkaloids, tannate of quinine, extracts of cina, of male fern, and of cubebs may be conveniently treated like resins. By rubbing them with three or four times their weight of sugar, and adding spirit of wine to make a thin electuary, they mix well with water. Without the addition of spirit these substances are apt to form a sediment which is very difficult to mix evenly by shaking.

Emulsions of Essential Oils, such as oil of turpentine, do not last long. They are best formed by brisk shaking with a thick mucilage. They require about ten times their weight of gum arabic or one yolk of egg to 5 to 10 grammes of ethereal oil. [One yolk will emulsify more if the operation is carefully done.—ED]

Camphor should be rubbed to a fine powder with the aid of a few drops of absolute alcohol, then mixed with ten times its weight of gum arabic or the yolk of an egg to 5 grammes (gum in preference), and the water added gradually. Any oil or balsam in the mixture should be mixed with the camphor before the gum is added. Syrup should be mixed up with the powder before the addition of water.

Phosphorus.—The preparation of this powerful medicine requires the greatest care. A mixture with a few atoms of the substance of the size of a pin's head may easily occasion fatal gastritis. It is, therefore, most important that when it is ordered in a mixture it should be perfectly divided. Some pharmacists have recommended the solution of phosphorus in hot mucilage. It is liable, however, in cooling to form small particles like wax, which makes this method highly dangerous. It should be dissolved in one hundred times its weight of almond or poppy oil in a test-tube by frequent dipping into hot water, and the oil solution emulsified in the proper way.

[The best plan to follow in such a case as this is to emulsify the proper quantity of the official ol. phosphori in the same manner as almond-oil is emulsified with acacia. Fortunately, emulsions of this kind are seldom ordered in this country.—ED.]

Wax, Spermaceti, and Cacao-butter are emulsified like the fixed oils. The wax is melted and poured into a hot mortar, the pestle also being heated. To 10 grammes of wax an equal weight of gum is added, and 15 grammes of hot water

N

are added gradually. After well mixing the mortar is partially cooled, and 85 grammes of cold water are stirred in gradually. Yellow wax should always be used for an emulsion. It gives a perfectly white emulsion. White wax cannot always be well emulsified, and the small proportion of tallow which it not infrequently contains is likely to impart to it a rancid taste.

[The rule may be safely laid down that fixed oils require the mortar and pestle, while volatile oils are better, as well as more quickly, emulsified by agitation. As volatile substances are generally required for immediate use—that is to say, the emulsions do not require to be kept for any length of time— a much smaller quantity of gum may be used than is here given. We have always used tragacanth in preference to ordinary gum, principally for the reason that a much smaller quantity is sufficient.—ED.]

INCE ON EMULSIONS.

MR. JOSEPH INCE thus speaks on this subject:—

Let the dispenser know when he has done his task, and when once he has formed his emulsion let him add rapidly the remaining ingredients. Many an emulsion is ruined by over-manipulation, and the oil having been incorporated is thrown out again by continuous stirring when mechanical mixture is concerned.

[Mr. William Gilmour of Edinburgh has lately made some experiments with a view to solving the query, Why should emulsions be stirred always in one direction? A theory has been propounded that by always stirring in one direction—for example, in the case of an oil emulsion, or in making cold cream—the oil is broken up in volume, minute globules resulting; but when the direction of stirring is reversed the oil tends to return to its original state. Mr. Gilmour had made various experiments, and found that, although a difference in the size of the globules was observable when examined by the microscope, little difference was apparent to the naked eye, and the two emulsions were, from a practical point of view, identical. It was noticed, however, that by stirring in two directions a little longer time was required to finish the emulsion, and this was the case with several oils when operated on with different emulsifying agents. On the whole, he considered that not much importance is to be attached to the theory of stirring one way, but it is advisable not to reverse the direction towards the end of the process, because at that point the tendency to spoil seems to be particularly marked.—ED.]

When liquids, limpid or viscous, are to be combined the very gentlest manipulation should be employed. Increase of pressure generates heat, and heat is fatal to union. Thus, when olive oil, mucilage, and water are to be emulsified, while care must be taken to have the three entirely under the control and action of the pestle, at the same time, lightness of hand cannot be too carefully studied.

On the other hand, when a solid has to be broken down and worked into a pasty saponaceous mass, an exactly opposite mode of treatment must be adopted. The object is to produce a kind of soap which can be only extemporaneously manufactured by strong, continued muscular action, with evolution of heat to complete the change.

Emulsions with Gum Arabic.—The slightest tendency of the mucilage to acidity will defeat the best manipulation. The Pharmacopœia directs 4 oz. of acacia to be dissolved in 6 oz. of distilled water. No heat should ever be resorted to to facilitate solution; and small picked gum arabic stirred occasionally in cold distilled water until the gum is dissolved gives a beautiful result. Powdered gum is a very foolish expedient for gaining time, and, when this mucilage is not bright without filtration, alteration of an injurious character may be anticipated. When finished, mucilage should be strained through muslin and kept in a cool place.

Ol. amygdal.	ʒiss.
Mucilag. gum. acac.	ʒiij.
Syrupi	ʒiss.
Aquæ dest.	ad ʒiij.

Put the whole of the mucilage into the mortar first; add the almond oil by degrees, but rapidly, with constant circular stirring in one direction, from left to right. Never add a second drop of oil until the first quantity has been emulsified. This is known by the creamy character of the product and its tendency to form clear spaces by leaving the sides of the mortar. Study two things—quickness of motion and lightness of hand. To the emulsion add the syrup and the water rapidly; of the latter, ½ oz. at a time. Five minutes should be employed in the whole operation. Slow dispensing is bad dispensing.

Powdered gum arabic is frequently ordered, and its exclusive use has been advocated by some Continental pharmacists.

Acaciæ pulv.	℈ij.
Ol. amygd.	ʒss.
Syrup. simpl.	ʒss.
Aquæ destillat.	ad ℥j.

Mix.

Add the whole of the powdered gum, and with a fair amount of force make it into a mucilage with 1½ drachm of water. Proceed as in the first case, lightness of hand being essential when once the mucilage is made. Six minutes should complete the operation; an experienced dispenser will want less, but these remarks throughout are written for beginners, and are not offered as advice to well-practised assistants.

Gum Resin Emulsions.—The mistura ferri composita will exemplify the subject. It is infinitely preferable to prepare it for stock in a concentrated form of four times the strength, and to keep the ferrous sulphate apart until required.

Myrrhæ	ʒss.
Sacchari	ʒss.
Potass. carb.	gr. xv.
Sp. myrist.	ʒij.
Aquæ rosæ	℥ixss.
Ferri sulphat.	gr. xij.

Beat the myrrh well, divide the beaten mass with the powdered sugar, and make into an emulsion with half the rosewater. Next add the carbonate of potash dissolved in the remainder of the water, and add the spirit last.

Recollect that potassium carbonate is a hostile ingredient in an emulsion when present with a second emulsifying agent. Proceeding in this way an excellent emulsion is produced in an extemporaneous manner; but there is a better mode.

Beat the myrrh as usual, divide with sugar, add the potash, and make a thick creamy emulsion with just sufficient water.

Let this stand, covered from the air, over night, and the following morning finish the operation. A few minutes' trituration will restore the whiteness, and such a mistura ferri will keep for some years without alteration.

Ammoniacum and asafœtida must both be converted into hydrated masses. Let them, before being manipulated, soak in a small quantity of water, when they are readily reduced to a pulpy condition, and form tolerable emulsions afterwards without any additional emulsifying agent.

Egg Emulsions require a skilful hand, and may be presented as permanent combinations. The first and last requisite is that the dispenser should abstain from the slightest mechanical force. Example :—

Ol. ricini	ʒj.
Vitelli ovi	j
Syrup. simpl.	ʒij.
Tinct. aurant.	ʒj.
Aquæ	ad ʒiij.

Break the egg-shell cleverly on the side-edge of a 2-oz. measure, into which let the albumen run. Entirely clear away the albumen (a fertile source of failure when this precaution is neglected). Keep the albumen to be used as liquid gum, and also for sugar-coating pills. Render the yolk (thrown into the mortar) perfectly smooth under the pestle with rapid circular motion; add the oil by degrees; if occasionally too thick, thin with a little water. Add the syrup next; then wash out the measure with a little water. Add the tincture last, and finally wash out the measure with the remaining water, and the process is complete.

Yolk of egg is supreme with regard to spermaceti, once a very favourite remedy with the accoucheur.

Cetacei	ʒj.
Vitelli ovi	½
Syrup. simpl.	ʒij.
Aquæ	ad ʒiss.

Break down the spermaceti; make it quite smooth in the syrup, then proceed as usual. All these egg emulsions keep.

When a dilute acid forms an ingredient in an emulsion, it should be added last, and there should be no fear of imperfect combination.

Copaiba Emulsions.—The practice has been recommended of making certain emulsions by very carefully smearing the bottle with the emulsifying agent. But it has been generally condemned, as not being an effectual mode. Copaiba forms an exception, and the balsam may be as well emulsified in this way as by any other.

Copaibæ	ʒvj.
Liq. potassæ	ʒiij.
Mucilag. acaciæ	℥j.
Sp. æther. nitr.	ʒiij.
Aq. cinnamom.	ad ℥viij.

Rotate the mucilage in the bottle, well covering the inside. Add the copaiba by degrees; perfectly emulsify by adding the alkali, previously diluted with 3 drachms of cinnamon-water; then the remainder of the cinnamon-water by degrees, retaining or allowing for 2 oz. with which to cleanse the measure from both the liquor potassæ and the spirit of nitrous ether, which should be added last.

Some prescribers are particular in the exhibition of copaiba, and occasionally want it to be taken without other ingredients. It can be so prepared, or made to combine at pleasure in all strengths by using freshly made thick mucilage ; thus :—

Pulv. gum. acaciæ	ʒj.
Aquæ destill.	ʒj.
Misce, et adde—	
Copaibæ	ʒiij.
Aquæ destill.	q.s. ad ℥iv.

Extractum filicis liquidum and tinctura cannabis Indicæ may both be made in the same manner.

NOTES.

Glycerine, like an alkaline salt, is a disturbing agent in an emulsion when another emulsifier is present. Many salts spoil emulsions when they are either neutral or acid, but when alkaline they favour the process. Borax has a beneficial action, and is in itself an excellent emulsifying agent.

Professor Redwood observes that mucilage answers better than an alkali for making an emulsion with castor oil or copaiba, but that the alkali is best for oil of almonds. Moreover, a good emulsion of oil of almonds and alkali is spoiled by the addition of mucilage. This Mr. Ince confirms from constant disappointment.

Milk makes a good emulsion with scammony, and is retained in official pharmacy for that purpose. Resin of jalap will not mix with milk, but will combine readily with almond emulsion.

M. Constantin (in 1854) advocated what may be called the ignition process for emulsion of the gum resins and resins. He took a weighed quantity of gum resin, and, having placed it in a mortar, added about four times its weight of alcohol. The spirit being ignited, the whole was triturated until all the alcohol was burned away. The gum resin became a soft extract; the liquid was then added in small quantities at a time, and a perfectly homogeneous emulsion was produced without subsequent separation. In the case of resins they must be converted into gum resins by the addition of powdered gum arabic. To the resin—balsam of tolu, for instance—twice its weight of gum arabic is to be added, and alcohol used in the same way. The peculiar taste and odour remain undiminished.

The method is expensive, but quite successful.

LOTIONS, LINIMENTS, AND INJECTIONS.

GENERALLY the same rules apply as to mixtures. Hager gives the following notes : Lead salts with tannin substances and with sulphates give heavy precipitates. With opium they cause a thick separation. Corrosive sublimate or nitrate of mercury solution likewise occasions a thick precipitate with opium, with mucilaginous or with albuminous substances. The prescriber ought to provide a means for keeping such precipitates in suspension. Mucilage of acacia will often answer. Camphor with a watery solution will separate, but with the addition of a little mucilage it is easily brought into suspension by shaking. Take the following prescription, quoted by Dr. Hager :—

					Grammes
Hydrarg. bichlor. corros.	.	.	.	.	1·0
Spirit. camphor.	.	.	.	.	.	30·0
Aquæ destill. .	.	.	.	.	.	300·0

M.   Ft. lotio.

Here a proper mixture will be made by dissolving the bichloride in 295 g. of water, mixing the camphor spirit with 5 g. of gum arabic in a little water, and then adding it to the sublimate solution. Of course, if this be done, the prescription should be so marked.

The suggestion to add mucilage of acacia to any lotion must be accepted with extreme caution, and every other method should be tried before resorting to it. The two mercurial lotions of our own Pharmacopœia are very good examples of the class referred to here, and no mucilage is considered necessary for suspending the precipitates. A 'shake-the-bottle' label should, of course, be appended. Sometimes a thickish precipitate may be to a great extent avoided by manipulation, as in the following case :—

Zinci sulph. .	.	.	.	.	.	.	gr. viij.
Tinct. lavand. co.		.	.	.	.	.	ʒij.
Spt. ròsmarini	.	.	.	.	.	.	ʒij.
Aquæ .	.	.	-	.	.	.	ad ℥viij.

Ft. lotio pro oculis.

Pour the tincture and spirit into the bottle containing 7 oz. of distilled water ; dissolve the sulphate of zinc in ½ oz. of water and add to the contents of the bottle. In this way there is comparatively little deposit. If spring-water of ordinary hardness be used there will be a copious deposit of carbonate of zinc and sulphate of lime.

Collyria are topical applications employed in the treatment of eye diseases ; in composition they do not differ from lotions. They are frequently applied by dropping into the eye ; when ordered, the dispenser should provide the patient with an eye-drop bottle, a small round bottle with a tube passing the cork. These bottles are extensively used at the London Ophthalmic Hospital. When half filled with fluid and held in the hand, tube downward, the fluid is forced out in drops by the expansion of the air caused by the heat of the hand. If the patient's circumstances do not warrant the supply of an eye-drop bottle, dispense in a blue-ribbed poison-bottle, and give a camel's-hair pencil for the application of the drops. When the pencil is applied, the inner surface of the upper eyelid should be touched, and not the eyeball. Solution of eserine is often called for as a remedy for the eyes. The solution becomes of a dark red colour, due to the formation of rubeserine. This, according to Mr. J. E. Saul, may be prevented by the addition of a very little sulphurous acid ; and as the red solution is apt to set up irritation, the means for preventing it should be brought under the notice of the prescriber. Cocaine solutions do not spoil if from ½ to 1 per cent. of boric acid is added to them, and the same applies to most alkaloids. The Pharmacopœia now orders camphor-water for the same purpose, but it is not so effectual, and has often given rise to local irritation.

The following is an example of intentional incompatibility :—

Plumbi diacet.	gr. iij.
Zinci sulph.	gr. iij.
Sp. vini rect.	℧ xx.
Aq. dest.	ad ℥iss.
Ft. collyrium.	

On compounding this a precipitate of sulphate of lead is formed.

Lotions similar to this are commonly used for old wounds, but less frequently for the eyes.

Lotions, like all preparations which are not intended to be swallowed, should be sent out in bottles different in shape from those used for mixtures. The labels should also be different.

In labelling a lotion a 'not-to-be-taken' label should be applied if it seem likely to be used as a mouth-wash, eye-drops, or injection. To use, as do some dispensers, an 'outward-application' label in all cases, is incorrect, and may possibly lead to a misunderstanding on the part of the patient.

LINIMENTS.

There are seldom great difficulties in this class of preparations. Lime-water to be mixed with oils should be added all at once, and well shaken. By adding gradually, a perfectly homogeneous combination is seldom attained.

The following are a few examples of exceptional difficulties The first is a hair-lotion of the character of a liniment :—

Liq. ammon.	℥j.
Ol. olivœ	℥j.
Paraffin. mollis	℥j.
Acet. canth.	℥ss.
Eau de Cologne	℥j.
Misce.	

By a slight modification of the formula, this may be compounded as follows :—

First add gradually the acetum cantharides to the spirits of hartshorn (use the liquor vol. cornu cervi and not liquor ammon. B.P.), constantly stirring with a glass rod until gas-bubbles no longer arise, then rub thoroughly well the paraffinum molle (use vaseline) with the oleum olivæ until a creamy compound is formed, afterwards gradually add little by little the partly neutralised liquor, constantly rubbing, adding lastly the eau de Cologne.

A favourite prescription with some medical men is a mixture of belladonna extract and liniment, such as the following :—

> Extract. belladonnæ . . . . . . ʒj.
> Liniment. belladon. . . . . . . ʒj.
> M. Ft. liniment.

It is the green extract which is here intended, and when it is rubbed up with the liniment there is an abundant separation of chlorophyll and extractive matter which cannot be avoided. Rub the extract in a mortar with ½ drachm of hot water ; then gradually add the liniment and strain through a small piece of calico. This is how the prescription is generally dispensed. The active principles are retained in solution. If the liniment is dispensed unstrained, the suspended matter attaches itself to the edges of the bottle. The following are similar cases which should be treated in the same way :—

> (a) Ext. belladonnæ . . ʒj.
> 　　Tinct. iodi . . . ʒiv.
> 　　Lin. camph. comp. ad ℥ij.
> 　　　M. Ft. lin.

> (b) Ext. belladonnæ . . ʒiss.
> 　　Lin. camph. co. . . ℥ij.
> 　　　M. Ft. lin.

In the case of (a), mix the tincture of iodine and liniment of camphor before adding to the thinned extract.

> Ext. belladonnæ . . . . . . ℥ij.
> Lin. ammoniæ . . . . ℥ij.
> M. Ft. lin.

Rub the extract with $\frac{1}{3}$ oz. of solution of ammonia, until solution is effected, then agitate with $1\frac{1}{3}$ oz. of olive-oil.

Ext. belladonnæ	. . . . . .	ʒij.
Ol. olivæ opt. .	. . . . . .	ʒij.

M. Ft. lin.

Thin the extract with hot water, and add the oil gradually. Do not strain.

HYPODERMIC INJECTIONS.

These have been introduced within the last twenty years, and are now in daily use by medical men. The syringes for them are of the capacity of 6, 10, and 20 minims, and the strength of solutions should be based upon minims, *not* fluid-grains.

Hypodermic injections should be perfectly clear, and the water for them should be pure distilled. Every vessel in which the injection is dispensed should be perfectly clean. Experience has pointed to the conclusion that when sores have resulted from hypodermic injections, these have been occasioned by some organic impurity in the water. Glycerine, if it form an ingredient in the injection, should be the purest procurable. Clear solutions may often require filtration, but it is important that the filters, before being used for the injection, should be thoroughly cleansed by passing a quantity of distilled water through them.

Cocaine Hydrochlorate gives the best results when used in solution not stronger than 5 per cent. Use only the cocaine which gives a crystalline precipitate when one drop of ammonia solution is added to a solution of the hydrochlorate (1 grain in 1 oz. of water).

Ergotin is always very acid in reaction, from the presence of acid phosphates of potash and lime ; this is partly the cause of the irritation and pustules which often follow its hypodermic injection. Mr. Gerrard proposes to neutralise it with ammonia, using the following formula : Take of—Ergotin, 10 grains, solution of ammonia, a sufficiency ; distilled water, to make 40 minims. Dissolve the ergotin in half the water, carefully neutralise with ammonia, then make up to 40 minims with water. If desired to be kept, 25 per cent. glycerine may be added. For the purpose of preservation we have had excellent results with chloral hydrate. Thymol is also one of the best preservatives for all kinds of hypodermic solutions. Take 1 grain of it in fine powder and agitate with 4 oz. of distilled water. This thymolated water is to be used in place of ordinary water. Carbolic acid is also effectual in the proportion of 5 or 10 minims to the ounce of distilled water. It does not give rise to irritation or constitutional effects, and, owing to its local anæsthetic action, it is believed by some medical men to be a beneficial addition to hypodermic injections.

INCOMPATIBLES.

MEDICAL MEN are but rarely good chemists, for this would necessitate longer devotion to chemistry than the average medical student can afford. Hence the importance of this branch being taken by the dispenser, in order that he may check the prescriber's combinations.

Many decompositions are intentional, such as in mist. ferri co., B.P., or in the frequent combination of tincture of opium with solution of subacetate of lead for injections; also in the following :—

> Ext. conii . . . . ℥ss.
> Liq. plumbi subacet. . . . . . ℥ss.
> Aquæ . . . . ad ℥vj.
> M. Ft. lot. Modo dicto utend.

In this case the abundant precipitate renders it almost creamy, and necessitates mixing half the water with the extract, and the remainder with the liquor before mixing, or a disagreeable lumpy mixture is produced. Such combinations may be dispensed as written, and sent out with a 'shake' label.

Occasionally, however, the decompositions are of such a character that the chemist may feel pretty sure that the writer of the prescription is unacquainted with the reaction, or has overlooked it. For example :—

> Sodæ sulphat. . . gr. xv. | Zinci sulphat. . . . ʒj.
> Potass. cit. . . . j. | Plumbi acet. . . . ʒij.
> M. Ft. pulv. Mitte vj. | M. Ft. pulv. Modo dict. utend.

In these cases metathesis takes place, the water of crystallisation of the sulphates is liberated, and the mass becomes wet. The use of an equivalent quantity of the dried salts removes the difficulty.

Prof. Remington gives the following in his 'Practice of Pharmacy' : —

Strychninæ sulph.	gr. j.
Potassii bromid.	ʒvii.
Aquæ q.s. ft.	ʒviii.

This solution deposits in a few hours the greater part of the strychnine salt as an insoluble bromide, which quickly subsides in transparent crystals. A lady in England lost her life by taking a similar mixture. She carefully refrained from shaking the bottle, the strychnine precipitated formed in the bottom, and in taking the last dose she swallowed nearly all of it.

One of the most remarkable cases of incompatibility is the following, which at first sight appears perfectly harmless, but at least one case of death is on record from the administration of a similar mixture :—

Potassæ chlorat.	ʒij.
Syr. ferri iodidi	ʒvj.
Vin. antim.	ʒss.
Æther. chlor.	ʒij.
Aq.	ad ʒviij.

This mixture is almost colourless when first prepared, but rapidly acquires a reddish-brown colour, and after a few days crystals of iodine are deposited. This is due to the action of chlorate of potash on ferrous iodide, the latter being oxidised by the former, chloride of potassium is produced, iodine set free, and, finally, ferric oxide or hydrate precipitated.

Incompatible mixtures are sometimes the result of impurities in the drugs used, thus :—

Sodæ hyposulph.	ʒj.
Acid. sulphuros.	ʒj.
Aq. rosæ	ad ʒviij.

The acid invariably contains some sulphuric acid, which throws out sulphur from the hyposulphite.

Acetate of Lead and *liquor plumbi subacetatis* are incompatible with infusion of opium, the vegetable astringents, soap, milk, or albumen. They are decomposed by sulphuric, hydrochloric, citric, and tartaric acids. Iodide of potassium causes a yellow precipitate, sulphuretted hydrogen a black precipitate, carbonated alkalies throw down a white, and the chromates of potash a lemon-yellow precipitate.

Alkaloids, whether alone or as salts, are nearly all precipitated from their solutions by tannic acid. They are, therefore, incompatible with this acid, and also with the various astringent vegetables containing it. Perchloride of mercury, Donovan's solution, free iodine, and double iodides generally also precipitate the alkaloids. (See Chapter on ' Quinine Mixtures.')

Almond Emulsion is separated by alcohol, tinctures, oxymel and syrup of squills, spirit of nitrous ether, hard water, and cream of tartar, which are more or less inimical to all emulsions.

Borax, powdered and rubbed up with mucilage, forms a soft powder like moist sugar, which cannot be made liquid by the addition of any further quantity of mucilage ; and acetate of lead, similarly treated, makes an opaque white jelly.

Calomel is decomposed by alkalies, alkaline earths and their carbonates, sulphides, hydrocyanic acid, bitter almonds, lime-water, iodide of potassium, iodine, soap, nitric acid, salts of iron, lead, and copper, nitrate of silver, &c. Be careful not to use *soap* in pills containing calomel.

Chlorides are incompatible with nitrate of silver, consequently bread containing common salt is an unsuitable excipient for pills of the nitrate.

Chloroform, if in a mixture containing opium or its preparations, will dissolve the narcotine, and, unless perfectly mixed, may cause an over-dose of this or some other alkaloid soluble in that vehicle to be given with the last dose.

A mixture containing liq. strychninæ, spt. ammon. arom., and spirit. chlorof. should have a 'shake' label placed upon it. A case has occurred where the chloroform was in part deposited and carried down with it in solution some of the strychnine which was set free by the ammonia.

Citrate of Potash.—

Potassæ cit.	.	.	℥iij.	Potassæ cit.	.	℥ij.
Potassæ bicarb.	.	℥ij.	Quininæ sulph.	.	gr. ix.
Tinct. aurant.	.	℥iv.	Aq.	.	ad ℥vj.
Aq.	.	ad ℥viij.			

Citrate of potash is rarely neutral; the sample used for the first prescription effervesced briskly with the bicarbonate, and examination proved the presence of nearly 5 per cent. of citric acid.

Another parcel was used for the second prescription, and a precipitate of quinine was produced: examination showed it to be alkaline. In each case the citrate should have been neutralised either with potassium carbonate or citric acid; but under any circumstance citrate of quinine will crystallise out of the second mixture.

The appearance of a sample of citrate of potash always indicates whether it is very acid or alkaline. If alkaline, it assumes a damp appearance and aggregates in lumps; but if acid, it seems dry and pulverulent.

Cochineal is precipitated by salts of zinc, bismuth, and nickel, in a lilac powder; iron gives a dark purple, tin a brilliant scarlet, and alumina the lakes.

Iodide of Potassium is decomposed by most acids and acidulous salts; this is really owing to the direct influence of sunlight. Oxidising acids, such as nitric acid, quickly liberate iodine; the others liberate hydriodic acid, which, under the influence of sunlight and in the presence of oxygen, is decomposed into iodine, the hydrogen going to form water. Most of the metallic salts decompose it. If iodide of potassium and spirit of nitrous ether are ordered in a mixture, the latter must be rendered slightly alkaline with bicarbonate of potash before it is used.

Bromide of Potassium is also, like the iodide, decomposed by acids.

Iron Salts.—A hydrated oxide or carbonate is generally thrown down by the alkalies and alkaline carbonates; Prussian blue is formed by ferrocyanide of potassium ; a precipitate of sulphide is yielded by sulphuretted hydrogen ; and tannin, and vegetable tinctures or infusions containing it, form with iron the basis of black ink.

The following is a good example of incompatibility :—

Potassii iodidi . . . . ʒiss.
Tr. ferri perchloridi . . . . . . ʒss.
Aquæ . . . . ad ʒvj.

Tinct. ferri perchloridi, indeed all non-scaled ferric salts, reduce iodide of potassium immediately on mixing solutions, free iodine being precipitated as a black sediment. The following equation explains the reaction :—

$$Fe_2Cl_6 + 2KI = 2FeCl_2 + 2KCl + I_2.$$

The mixture is a most dangerous combination, and should never be dispensed.

Nitrate of Potash is decomposed by most of the sulphates, and forms a double salt with alum.

Solution of Potash and other alkalies are incompatible with acids, ammonia salts, calomel, iodides, and with vegetable infusions containing an alkaloid principle.

Strychnine is precipitated from solution of its salts by alkalies and their carbonates. Liq. strychninæ and liq. arsenicalis are sometimes prescribed together. In this form the alkali of the latter precipitates the strychnine, so that a ' shake-the-bottle' label must be used. If an opportunity occur, the dispenser should advise the prescriber to use liq. arsenic, hydrochloricus, giving the reason for so doing.

In a paper by Mr. Henry Campbell on incompatibilities (*The Chemist and Druggist*, April 28, 1888, page 561), it is pointed out that, although bicarbonate of soda is generally considered to be incompatible with *liquor strychninæ*, it does not follow that the strychnine will always be precipitated ; the following mixture, for example, remains clear :—

Liquoris strychninæ . . . . . ♏ v.
Sodii bicarbonatis . . . . . gr. xv,
Aquæ . . . . . . ad ʒj.

The dose of the strychnine solution contains $\frac{1}{32}$ grain of alkaloid, forming in the ounce mixture a solution of the strength of 1 in 9,600, while the solubility of the alkaloid in water is about 1 in 5,700.

The same writer points out that the reaction between iodide of potassium and solution of strychnine is considerably retarded by the addition of tragacanth mucilage.

BRIEF SUMMARY OF INCOMPATIBILITIES.

Acid arsenious, with lime-water, oxide of iron, magnesia.

Acids generally, with alkalies, acetates, metallic oxides.

Albumen, with acids, spirit, tannin, corrosive sublimate.

Alkaloidal salts generally, with tannin, alkaline and earthy carbonates, iodine and its compounds, liquorice, strong mucilages, alkaline and ammoniated tinctures.

Alum sulphate with alkalies and alkaline carbonates.

Ammonium bromide, with mineral acids, alkaline carbonates, chlorine, chlorate and bichromate of potash, nitrate of silver, calomel.

Apomorphine (hydrochlorate), with carbonate and bicarbonate of soda, salts of iron, iodine, and tannin.

Barium chloride, with sulphuric and phosphoric acids and their salts, tartrates and carbonates, medicinal wines and vegetable infusions.

Bicarbonate of soda, with acids, tannin, salts of the metals and of the alkaloids.

Bismuth subnitrate, with tannin, sulphur, sulphide of antimony, calomel.

Chloral hydrate, with water (slow decomposition), warm water, alkaline carbonates, vegetable alkalies, ammonia salts, nitrate of mercury, calomel. ·

Chlorate of potash, with mineral acids, organic substances, sulphur, carbon, calomel, iodide of iron, &c.

Chlorine (chlorine-water), with alkalies, alkaline carbonates, salts of ammonia, vegetable salts, nitrate of silver, lead salts, tannin, vegetable mucilages, extracts, waters, infusions, tinctures and syrups, milk, and emulsions.

Corrosive sublimate, with carbonates, lime-water, iodide of potassium, opium, vegetable infusions, tannin, but compatible with the carbonates of lime, baryta, and strontia, either in powder or super-carbonated solution.

Digitalis, with tannin, sugar of lead, iodine, iodide of potassium, alkaline carbonates.

Golden sulphuret of antimony, with bicarbonate of soda, cream of tartar, calomel, subnitrate of bismuth.

Gum arabic, with perchloride of iron, lead salts, spirit, ethereal tinctures, borax.

Iodine, with ammonia, starch, metallic salts, fatty or essential oils, emulsions, chloral, earthy carbonates, gum arabic, tragacanth, salep.

Iron powdered (iron reduced by hydrogen) with aloes, vegetable infusions and extracts, tannin, metallic and alkaloidal salts.

Iron salts, with alkaline carbonates, vegetable infusions and extracts, tannin, mucilage.

Lime-water, with acids, carbonates, ammonia salts, metallic salts, tartrates, infusions, tinctures, tannin.

Morphine and its salts, with oxide of iron, salts of iron, manganese, and silver.

Musk, with acids, acetates, tannin, ergot of rye, metallic salts.

Nitrate of silver, with hydrochloric, sulphuric, acetic, and tartaric acids and their salts, hydrocyanic acid and its compounds, iodine, iodide and bromide of potassium, alkaline and earthy carbonates, sulphur, and sulphide of antimony.

Nitrite of amyl, with tinctures, alkaline carbonates, calomel, lead salts, proto-salts of iron, iodide of potassium.

Opium, with alkaline carbonates, salts of the metals, tannin, iodine, chlorine-water, and nux vomica. Although opium and belladonna are supposed to be physiologically incompatible, they are often administered together with good results.

Pepsin, with alcohol, tinctures.

Permanganate of potash, with organic substances.

Salicylic acid and salicylate of soda, with iron salts, iodide of potassium, lime-water.

Strophanthus (tincture) in water undergoes hydrolysis, with formation of a toxic substance.

Tannin, with mucilage, all metallic salts, lime-water, alkaline carbonates and bicarbonates, egg albumen, gelatine.

Tartar emetic, with acids, alkalies, soap, calomel, tannin, rhubarb, cinchona, gum arabic, opium.

DISPENSING OF INCOMPATIBLES.

It is not easy to lay down any rule for the dispenser when he comes across a case of incompatibility. In such cases he would do well to put to himself, previous to compounding the prescription, such questions as the following :—(1) Was this incompatibility foreseen and intended by the prescriber? (2) Does it in any way endanger the health of the patient? (3) Is it necessary to trouble the prescriber (supposing he can be communicated with) regarding the incompatibility? (4) Can the incompatibility be in any way mitigated or avoided? The subjoined cases are given as illustrations of these remarks :—

Magnes. carb. .	ʒij.
Acid. sulph. dil.	ʒiss.
Magnes. sulph. .	ʒiss.
Quininæ sulph. ..	ʒss.
Aq. menth. pip.	ad ʒiv.

Now, as sulphate of magnesia is already ordered in the prescription, it is improbable that the prescriber intended also the addition of this salt by extemporaneous preparation. Further, the prescriber probably adds the acid merely to assist the solution of the quinine, and, although it is added in excess in this instance, it is generally so added in quinine mixtures. Lastly, there is the probability that the magnesia carbonate was intended to act as an antacid ; so that, everything considered, there was no difficulty in substituting q. s. of acid to dissolve the quinine for ʒiss. On the whole, however, it is better to omit the acid altogether, because the soluble sulphate of quinine will be decomposed by the magnesia carbonate. It answers well to rub the quinine to fine powder and suspend in the mixture along with the carbonate.

Potass. iodid.	.	.	.	.	.	.	ʒiss.
Nepenthe .	.	.	.	.	.	.	ʒiss.
Ammon. carb.	.	.	.	.	.	.	ʒj.
Acid. phosph. dil.	.	.	.	.	.	.	℥ss.
Syr. tolutan.	.	.	.	.	.	.	℥j.
Aq. camph.	.	.	.	.	.	.	ad ℥viij.

It is not easy to arrive at any satisfactory conclusion as to the intention of the prescriber in this instance ; but as the phosphate of ammonia formed is altogether harmless, and as free phosphoric acid in the mixture would liberate iodine and precipitate the alkaloid of the nepenthe, there was no hesitation in dispensing the prescription as it stood.

Mucilag. acac.	.	.	.	.	.	.	ʒj.
Sodæ hyposulphit.	.	.	.	.	.	.	ʒiv.
Ol. menth. pip.	.	.	.	.	.	.	♏ xij.
Liq. bismuthi (B.P. 1867) .	.	.	. .	.	ʒiss.
Liq. morph. hydrochlor.	.	.	.	.	.	ʒij.
Aq.	.	.	.	.	.	.	ad ℥vj.

This will probably appear a very innocent mixture when first dispensed, but if prepared strictly according to the letter it will almost certainly bring the dispenser into trouble. It will form a clear mixture when first dispensed, but after an interval, depending on the purity of the ingredients, it will turn first brown and then quite black, and become quite unfit for use. A prescription such as this should never be dispensed without an explanation to the patient of the changes which may be expected to take place, and a caution not to use the mixture after decomposition. Decomposition will be retarded if an equivalent be added of pure gum arabic instead of mucilage, and of pure muriate of morphine instead of the official solution, and, above all, if the solution of bismuth be rendered decidedly alkaline.

The following is a prescription which was given by the Illinois State Board of Pharmacy at an examination :—

(1) Tinct. ferri mur.	ʒij.
(2) Sp. æther. nitric.	ʒss.
(3) Mucilag. acaciæ	ʒj.
Syrup q.s. (i.e. 10 drachms) ut ft. . .	ʒiij.

It is, in the ordinary sense of the term, incompatible, but Mr. Joseph Ince, commenting upon it, says that, made most ways, it assumes the form of a thick jelly, which may be sent out in a covered pot. Reason thus :—Here are three ingredients likely to react upon each other, of which mucilage is chief. There are 10 drachms of protective agent (syrup) at disposal ; divide it into ʒij. with the tincture, ʒiij. with the spirit of nitrous ether, and ʒv. with mucilage, which wants it most.

(1) Tinct. ferri mur.	ʒij.
Syrupi	ʒij.

M.

(2) Sp. æther. nitr.	ʒss.
Syrupi.	ʒiij.

M.

(3) Mucilag. acaciæ	ʒj.
Syrupi	ʒv.

M.

Combine the three solutions, and a beautiful preparation is the result.

The same commentator produces a black lotion from the following :—

Hydrarg. submur.	gr. iij.
Zinci chlorid.	gr. iij.
Aq. calcis	ʒj.

The method adopted was to make the black wash first, then to add the zinc chloride. But nature would have her own way : in the course of a few hours the zinc chloride interacts with the mercurous oxide, and the lotion becomes white. It is therefore just as well to add the zinc chloride to the lime-water in the first instance.

The following is given by Mr. Campbell. It shows how the order of mixing affects the result.

Liquoris hydrargyri perchloridi	.	.	.	ʒj.
Ammoniæ carbonatis	.	.	.	.	gr. v.
Potassii iodidi	.	.	.	.	.	gr. v.
Aquæ .	.	.	.	.	.	.	ad ʒj.

Although an alkaline carbonate orms a precipitate with mercuric chloride, still, if in the above mixture the first and third ingredients be mixed, and the solution of the carbonate then added, no precipitate occurs. It common water be used, a slight precipitate of calcium carbonate forms, but it is free from mercury.

Other instances of incompatibility have been given under Mixtures, Pills, etc.

EXPLOSIVE AND INFLAMMABLE COMPOUNDS.

Whenever substances rich in oxygen, or easily deoxidised, are ordered to be mixed with other ingredients, the dispenser should always carefully consider the order of mixing. Such substances should never be rubbed with easily-oxidisable bodies.

Substances which easily part with their oxygen are picric acid, and chlorate, iodate, bichromate, permanganate, nitrate, and picrate of potash, nitrate and oxide of silver, chlorate of calcium, &c. Such substances should be first rubbed to a powder in a mortar. They should then be mixed with the safe ingredients, and lightly stirred with a wooden rod with the easily-oxidisable substances. Of the latter may be named charcoal, organic powders, iodine, sulphur, sulphides, reduced iron, powdered iron, iodide of iron, hypophosphite of calcium, camphor, ethereal oils, and ammonia salts.

The following are specimens of explosive compounds :—

							Parts
Potass. chlorat. .	.	.	.	.	.	.	2·0
Lactis sulphuris .	.	.	.	.	.	.	3·0
Antim. sulph. aur.	.	.	.	.	.	.	0·5
Zinci valerianatis	.	.	.	.	.	.	0·5
Sacchari .	.	.	.	.	.	. .	5·0

M. Ft. pulv. Divide in partes 20 æquales.

The chlorate of potash should first be rubbed to a fine powder ; the other ingredients should be separately mixed ; lastly, the chlorate should be combined with the other mixture by stirring with a quill. The pressure of a pestle would ensure a dangerous detonation—indeed, chlorates are amongst the most explosive compounds known, and should always be handled carefully.

The same applies to hypophosphites—never rub them too hard, and be careful how you apply heat to them, either when dry or in solution, especially with glycerine.

Oxide of Silver, if to be combined with any organic substance, should be first damped with water. If creosote is ordered with oxide of silver in a pill, it will explode. Pills containing oxide of silver are liable to inflame if they become warm. They have taken fire in the pocket of a customer, causing severe burns. The results of many, and most, unsafe experiments, which we would advise no young dispenser to reproduce, lead to one satisfactory method of proceeding in cases like that of oxide of silver. When it is a question of an explosive salt, or one that under any circumstance may become explosive, dilute it first, and separately, with twice its weight of a neutral excipient. Make into a protected mass the remaining explosive ingredient. Take, for example, the pill with oxide of silver and creosote, such as :—

	Argenti oxid.	.	.	.	.	.	.	gr. vj.
	Creosoti	.	.	.	.	.	.	gtt. vj.
M.	Ft. pil. vj.							

Proceed as follows :—

	Argenti oxid.	.	.	.	.	.	.	gr. vj.
	Pulv. glycyrrh.	.	.	.	.	.	.	gr. xij.
M.								
	Creosoti	.	.	.	.	.	.	gtt. vj.
	Saponis .	.	.	.	.	.	.	gr. vj.
M.	Ft. massa.							

Add the first to the second, and mass with mucilage.

This system, varied according to formula, has been practised successfully under even more perilous conditions. With metallic oxides, except zinc oxide, use glycerine or mucilage ; never a reducing agent or one containing an excess of carbon, such as syrup, honey, and the like.

Nitrogen Compounds.—Tincture of iodine and ammonia are often prescribed together, and iodide of nitrogen is produced under certain conditions. An explosion has resulted from the preparation of the following prescription, iodide of nitrogen being evidently the cause :—

Iodi .	.	.	.	.	.	.	ʒij.
Lin. camph. co.	.	.	.	.	.	.	ℨj.
Lin. saponis co.	.	.	.	..	.	.	℥j.

A concentrated solution of iodine and iodide of potassium was filtered through paper. The next day the filter was touched with a view to being removed, when the paper and funnel were shivered into atoms with a loud explosion.

Bismuth subnitrate and bicarbonate of soda or potash in a mixture frequently cause an explosion, owing to the interaction of the two salts. Instances have already been given of mixtures exhibiting this reaction.

Tinct. ferri perchloridi, B.P., with an equal quantity of acid. nitrohydrochlor. dil., develops sufficient gas to burst the bottle.

Chloral hydrate and spt. ammon. arom. dispensed together in mixture, and allowed to stand for a few hours well corked, result in an explosion, due to the alkali decomposing the chloral hydrate with liberation of chloroform.

DISPENSING FOREIGN PRESCRIPTIONS.

IN seaport towns, health-resorts, and cities with considerable foreign colonies, chemists are, no doubt, frequently called upon to dispense prescriptions of foreign origin. But it possibly happens sometimes that, owing to want of the necessary initiation into the not very formidable intricacies of foreign dispensing, customers are told that the prescription they have presented for dispensing, being a foreign one, cannot be made out. The consequence, probably, is that the customer goes and gets elsewhere that which, if he was only aware of it, the chemist who turns him away has an abundance of on his own shelves. In this chapter such information regarding French and German methods of dispensing is given as will assist in the compounding of continental prescriptions. In the appendix will be found a table of terms likely to occur in French and German prescriptions.

GERMAN PRESCRIPTIONS.

The most confusing thing about German prescriptions is the chemical nomenclature, of which the following is a fair example :—

| Kali hydrojodici | . | . | . | . | . | . | 6,0 |
| Aquæ depuratæ | . | . | . | . | . | . 180,0 |

Rendered into Anglo-Latin, this is :—

| Potassii iodidi | . | . | . | . | . | . ℈iss. } nearly |
| Aquæ destillatæ | . | . | . | . | . | . ℥vj. |

In dealing with German prescriptions the difficulty of the nomenclature, independently of minor grammatical differences, resolves itself into acquiring the English terms for a limited number of drugs and preparations. The use of the adjective is, perhaps, the most striking deviation from the Anglo-Latin nomenclature. Thus, for *ferrum sulphuricum* we should read, according to English custom, ferri sulphas ; for *ferrum iodatum*, ferri iodidum, and so on. With the exception of particular instances mentioned hereafter, nearly everything will, with a very little thought, be self-evident to the dispenser sufficiently well up in his Latin not to fall into the error attributed to an American *confrère*, who sent to his wholesale house for a supply of 'aqua fervida.' There still exist, however, in various parts of the Continent, medical men of the old school, who, in addition to prescribing by the old grain, drachm, and ounce system, make use of some of the cabalistic signs handed down to us from past generations. Four of these are met with as abbreviations rather frequently, viz. : ℥ for pulvis, V for aqua, ♯ for saccharum, and ℥ for spiritus. These gentlemen also prefer using obsolete terms for well-known preparations.

The following are most frequently met with :—

For Acetum plumbi	*read* Liq. plumbi subacet.
,, ,, saturninum	,, ,, ,,
,, Aqua saturni	,, ,, ,, dilutus
,, ,, phagædenica	,, Lotio hydrargyri flava
,, ,, fontana	,, Aqua pura
,, Aquila alba	,, Hydrargyri subchloridum
,, Deutojoduretum hydrargyri	,, ,, iodid. rubrum
,, Flores benzoës	,, Acidum benzoicum
,, ,, naphæ	,, Flores aurantii
,, ,, zinci	,, Zinci oxidum
,, Gummi mimosæ	,, Gummi acaciæ
,, Lapis infernalis	,, Argenti nitras
,, Magisterium bismuthi	,, Bismuthi subnitras
,, Mercurius	,, Hydrargyrum
,, Natrum carbonicum acidulum	,, Sodæ bicarbonas
,, Natro-kali tartaricum	,, Soda tartarata
,, Nihilum album	,, Zinci oxidum
,, Oleum anthos	,, Oleum rosmarini

For Oleum de cedro	*read* Oleum limonis
,, Protojoduretum hydrargyri	,, Hydrarg. iodid. viride
,, Pulvis Kurellæ	,, Pulv. glycrrh. comp.
,, Saccharum saturni	,, Plumbi acetas
,, Sal amarum	,, Magnesiæ sulphas
,, ,, mirabile	,, Sodæ sulphas
,, Sapo viridis	,, Sapo mollis
,, Syrupus diacodii	,, Syr. papav. alb.
,, Spiritus Mindereri	,, Liq. ammon. acet.
,, Tinctura thebaica	,, Tinct. opii

More modern deviations from the Anglo-Latin nomen-clature are given below, those adopted by the Pharmacopœa Germanica having the prefix P.G. :—

For Acidum phenylicum	*read* Acid carbolic
,, P.G. Aqua amygdalarum amararum	,, Aq. lauro-cerasi
,, P.G. Calcaria usta	,, Calx
,, P.G. Cortex chinæ	,, Cinchona
,, P.G. Chininum	,, Quinina
,, P.G. Flores cinæ	,, Santonica
,, P.G. Gutti	,, Cambogia
,, Hydrargyrum amidato-bichlorat	,, Hydrarg. ammoniat.
,, P.G. Kalium	,, Potassium.
,, P.G. Kali	,, Potassa
,, Linimentum volatile	,, Linim. ammoniæ
,, P.G. Radix liquiritiæ	,, Glycyrrhiza
,, P.G. Liquor ammonii caustici	,, Liq. ammoniæ
,, P.G. Natrium	,, Sodium
,, P.G. Natrum	,, Soda
,, P.G. Stibium	,, Antimonium
,, P.G. Semen strychni	,, Nux vomica
,, Sulfur auratum	,, Antimon. sulphurat.
,, P.G. Tartarus depuratus	,, Potass. bitartras
,, P.G. ,, natronatus	,, Soda tartarata
,, P.G. ,, stibiatus	,, Antimon. tartarat.
,, P.G. Tinct. opii benzoica	,, Tinct. camph. co.
,, P.G. Unguent. paraffini	,, Paraffinum molle
,, P.G. Vinum stibiatum	,, Vin. antimoniale

Preparations peculiar to German pharmacy which will require reference to the German Pharmacopœia, or some other text-book, such as Hager's 'Manuale Pharmaceuticum,' are :—

Ammonium chloratum ferratum (Ammon. muriatico-ferratum)
Aqua chlorata (Liq. chlori)
Elixir aurantiorum comp.
Elixir e succo liquiritiæ (Elixir pectorale)
Elixir proprietatis (Paracelsi)
Ferrum aceticum (liq. and tinct.)
Ferrum pomatum (ext. and tinct.)
Liq. ammon. anisatus
Liq. aluminii acetici
Linimentum saponato-camph.
Mixtura sulfurica acida (Elixir acidum Halleri)
Mixtura oleoso-balsamica (Balsamum-vitæ Hoffmani)
Mucilago salep

Oleum hyosciami coctum
Sal thermarum carolinensium (Sal carolinum factitium)
Sapo jalapinus
Species pectorales
Species laxantes (St. Germain)
Species lignorum
Spiritus formicarum
Spir. saponis
Tinctura amara
Tinctura lignorum
Tinct. ferri chlorati ætherea (Tinct. nervina Bestuscheffii)
Tinctura opii crocata (Laudanum liquidum Sydenhami)
Unguent. Hebræ
Vinum aromaticum

The above have been selected as being what may be called of every-day occurrence, and, although a knowledge of them does not constitute all that is required of a German dispenser quite *au fait* with his work, it will help to clear away many *primâ-facie* difficulties.

All quantities ordered are understood to be by weight, fluid measures not being countenanced by the German authorities. The minim is still very frequently represented by the drop (gutta), of which 20 are considered equal to 1 gramme. As drops vary materially according to the density of the fluid and the size of the bottle, this is very unsatisfactory. The tare of the dispensing-bottle being taken, the various ingredients ordered on the prescription are successively weighed into it, commencing with the smallest quantities and finishing with the vehicle. For this purpose English bottles may be said to hold 30 grammes or more per oz. capacity of water, and denser fluids respectively, or 24 grammes of spirit or tinctures.

The very convenient way of prescribing the vehicle, *ad* so many ounces, is adopted by but few foreign physicians, and the few who do so have mostly practised some time in this country.

As in England, mixtures predominate in German prescribing. Solutions of extracts (such as ext. taraxaci, trifolii,

graminis, &c.), decoctions and infusions, and oil or seed emulsions occur, however, somewhat more frequently. Decoctions
and infusions are directed to be recently prepared, and, if
definite proportions are not indicated by the prescriber, are to
be made in the proportion of 1 in 10. Seed emulsions, prepared from almonds, poppy, hemp, or henbane seeds, also
1 in 10, or obtained by crushing the seeds, with the addition
of a little water, in a metal mortar, until a pasty, homogeneous
mass is produced, to which the bulk of the water is gradually
added, and the resulting milky fluid strained through flannel.
Oil emulsions are, according to the Ph. Germ., directed to be
made of oil 2, gum acaciæ 1, and water 17 parts.

The Potio Riveri of the Ph. Germ. is a fair type of what are
called 'saturations,' i.e., an alkaline carbonate saturated with
an organic acid (preferably acetic or citric), the carbonic acid
evolved being partly absorbed by the vehicle.

Draughts, in the strict application of the term, are almost
unknown. Drops, however, are a favourite form of administering medicines. They usually consist of tinctures or a solution of extract, alkaloid, &c.

Pills are not, perhaps, quite so much in vogue as in
England, but large quantities are sometimes prescribed, 120,
or even 360, being ordered for one patient. Pill-machines
being made to cut 30, that number or its multiples are generally ordered. Their weight scarcely ever exceeds 2 grains,
4 or 5 grain pills being quite the exception. Lycopodium
is very generally employed to roll the pills in, unless some
other powder, such as p. cinnamomi, is specially prescribed,
and gold and silver coating is sometimes directed for better-
class patients.

Powders to the number of 12, 16, 24, or 48 are also much
in request. When not directed to be divided off into doses
they are dispensed in bulk, to be taken by the teaspoonful; in
the latter case they are ordered 'ad scatulam,' or, if they
contain elœosacchara, narcotic extracts, camphor, musk, or
other volatile substances, 'ad vitrum.' Extracts to be incorporated with powders are kept as 'extracta sicca,' containing

equal parts of extract and pulv. glycyrrh. Elœosacchara are mixtures consisting of 1 drop of essential oil to 2 grammes of sugar. Volatile substances, when ordered in powders divided off into doses, are ordered 'in charta cerata,' *i.e.*, waxed paper. Either the dose for each powder is prescribed, with the direction 'dentur tales doses No. X.,' or the ingredients for a number are ordered in the aggregate, with an intimation to 'divide in partes æquales No. X.'

Ointments are much of the same nature as here, and do not call for any particular remarks. . Ungt. hydr. fort. is occasionally prescribed, weighed off in quantities from 1 to 4 grammes, to be wrapped up separately in waxed paper to the number of 12 to 20.

Plasters are sometimes ordered in bulk for the patient to spread them himself. Empl. vesicatorium stands for empl. cantharidis.

Directions for use are invariably written in German, certain abbreviations being made use of, *e.g.*, 3 tgl. 1 Essl.= Dreimal täglich einen Esslöffelvoll, *i.e.*, one tablespoonful three times daily ('to be taken' being understood); 2 stl. 1 Theel=Zweistündlich einen Theelöffelvoll, *i.e.*, a teaspoonful every two hours. The following words occur constantly :—

Esslöffelvoll	= tablespoonful	Pillen	= pills
Theelöffelvoll	= teaspoonful	Pulver	= powder
Kaffeelöffelvoll	= ditto	Ausserlich	= for external use
Kinderlöffelvoll	= dessertspoonful	Morgens	= in the morning
Tropfen	= drops	Abends	= in the evening
Einreibung	= embrocation	In Wasser	= in water
Einspritzung	= injection	Auf Zucker	= on sugar
Umschlag	= lotion	Zu nehmen	= to be taken
Salbe	= ointment	Umgeschüttelt	= to be shaken

When prescribing doses of the more active substances in excess of the Pharmacopœia maxima the physician adds a note of exclamation after the weight (thus : morph. acet., 0,5 !), to indicate that he is well aware of the fact and takes the responsibility on himself.

The word 'cito!' or even 'citissime' is sometimes added, to signify to the dispenser that the prescription is to be dispensed immediately, as the patient is probably endangered if delayed.

Facsimile Prescriptions.—The difficulties of nomenclature over, the dispenser has now to face the handwriting of German prescriptions, which differs materially from English handwriting. A knowledge of this can only be acquired by practice with the originals, of which we submit a few that will be found useful for exercise and reference. It may surprise English dispensers to learn that these are selected rather for purposes of illustration than as being particularly difficult ones, though one or two present some hard nuts to crack. We add the correct reading of and occasional comments on these prescriptions :—

Rp. Apomorph. mur. cryst.	.	.	0·04 ($\frac{2}{3}$ gr.)
Morph. mur.	.	.	0·02 ($\frac{3}{10}$ gr.)
Aquæ amygd. amar. .	.	.	5·0 (77 grs.)
Elix. pector.	.	.	20·0 ($\frac{1}{2}$ oz. av. 85 grs.)
Aqu. destill.	.	.	30·0 (1 oz. av. 25 grs.)
Syr. simpl..	.	.	15·0 ($\frac{1}{2}$ oz. av. 13 grs.)

M. D. S. 4 mal täglich einen Theelöffelvoll.

In this prescription the quantities are, as usual, given in metric weights. The liquids, as well as the solids, should be weighed into the bottle, which by preference should be of black glass, in order to prevent decomposition of the apomorphine.

The aq. amygd. amar. of the prescription is the aqua laurocerasi, and elixir pectorale is the elixir e succo liquirit. of the German Pharmacopœia.

The directions mean 'four times daily one teaspoonful.'

The mark 1·45 in the margin means that the price charged was 1 mark 45 pfennige=1*s.* 5*d.* The price is regulated in Germany by a Government tariff which the pharmacist may not exceed under penalty of a heavy fine.

Chinini muriat.　.　.　.　.　.　.　1·0
Aqu. dest.　.　.　.　.　.　.　30·0
Acid. muriat. dil.　.　.　.　.　.　q.s.
S. Nachmittags einen Esslöffelvoll.

This is quoted chiefly for the directions, which are rather unusual, namely, a tablespoonful in the afternoon.

| Iodoform | . | . | . | 3·0 | Vasel. alb. . | . | . | 10·0 |
| Ungt. cerei | . | . | . | 10.0 | Cumarin | . | . .. | 0·4 |

M. Ft. ungt. D. S. Mgs. (Morgens) einzureiben.

An ointment 'to be rubbed in, in the morning.' The ung. cerei is composed of olive oil 7 parts and yellow wax 3 parts. The letters on the margin—'o. a. e. l.'—stand for 'olla alba epistomio ligneo'—a white jar with wooden top. Price charged, 1m. 30pf.

Rp. Tinct. chinæ comp. . . . . . .
  ,,   valer. æther. . . . . . . a. ʒij.

M. D. S. Alle 2 Stunden, 15 Tropfen auf Zucker.

This is written by one of the old-fashioned doctors who still use the old measures. The directions mean 'fifteen drops on sugar every two hours.' Observe the word 'cito' at the end o the prescription as an injunction to the dispenser.

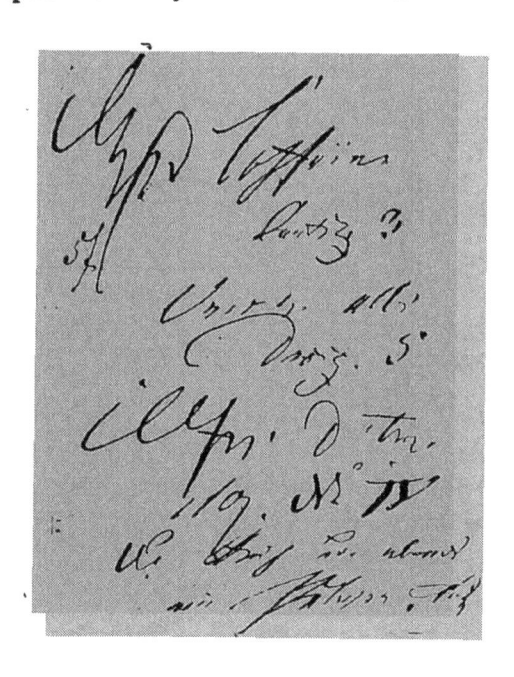

Rp. Coffeini . . . . . . centig. 3
  Sacch. albi . . . . . decig. 5

M. Ft. pulv., d. tales dos. No. IV. S. Morg. und Abends ein Pulver.

This prescriber looks like taking first prize for bad writing in this competition. 'Caffeine' in English is 'coffein' in German. The doctor's peculiar care to write out 'centig.' and 'decig.' assists marvellously to obscure his prescription for foreign readers. Price charged, 50pf.=6*d*.

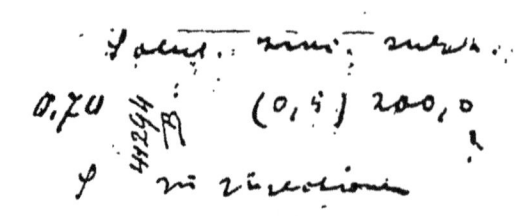

Rp. Tinct. rhei vinos. . . . . . . 6·00
    ,,   valcr. . . . . 4·00
  Elix. aur. comp. , ... 8·00
D. S. Zweimal täglich, 18–20 T.

Vinous tincture of rhubarb is made of rhubarb 8, orange-peel 2, cardamoms 1, and sherry 100 parts. The directions are given here very curtly, but no doubt mean '18 to 20 drops twice daily.' Price charged, 0·85pf.=10*d*.

Solut. zinci sulph. (0·5) . . . . . 200·0
S. pro injectione.

This is simple enough. Half a gramme of sulphate of zinc to be dissolved in 200 grammes of water.

Camf. trit. . . . . 3j.
Tere c.
    Mucil. g. arab. . . . . 3iv.
    Laud. liq. Syd. . . . . . . 3ij.
    Syr. ♯ . . . . 3vj.
    V. dest. . . . . 3vj.

D. S. Morgens und Abends einen Esslöffelvoll.

In this prescription we come across the old Arabic signs
for sugar and water. The directions mean 'one tablespoonful
night and morning.'

[handwritten prescription facsimile]

Chinini sulfuric . . . . . . gram. 2
Extract. valerian. . . . . . gram. 4
Extract. tarax. . . . . . . q.s.

Ut f. pilul. No. 60. Conspergentur pulv. cass. cinnam. D. S.
Dreimal täglich vier Pille zu nehmen.

The only point about this prescription which needs explanation is the interpolation of the dispenser, who found that 1
gramme extract. tarax. and 5 grammes of an inert substance,
for which he chose pulv. rad. althææ, were required to make
the mass. The pills were rolled in pulv. cinnamom.

Iod. pur. . . . . 0·5
Kalii iodat. . . . . 2·0
Ungt. paraff. . . . . 20·0
F. ungt.   D. S.

It is hardly necessary to say that for 'kalii iodat.' iodide of potassium is intended, and paraffinum molle for 'ungt. paraff.' On the margin the dispenser has run out the calculation of his charge as by law allowed. The first three figures are for the ingredients, the last for the vessel, and the others for the mixing and the labelling, &c., making 1*s*. 1*d*. in all. The 'o. gris.' means the ointment was dispensed in an earthenware pot— *olla grisea*.

FRENCH PRESCRIPTIONS.

The art of dispensing 'as in France' is fairly told in the following article, written by a French pharmacien, who bases his remarks upon a week's work, which consisted of 33 potions (mixtures), 1 suppository, 9 powders, 5 drops, 5 solutés (solutions), 1 inhalation, 4 collutoires (collutoria), 9 pommades (ointments), 10 syrups, 3 hypodermic injections, 7 cachets, 4 liniments, 3 pills, 2 wines, and 4 mélanges.

The Codex gives some general directions to be observed in the preparation of potions. All powders, vegetable or mineral, it directs, should be divided by the syrup or gum which may be prescribed. Kermes mineral, which is frequently occurring, should be well triturated with sugar before the addition of the other ingredients, and all volatile substances, such as ethers, should be added last. The first prescription containing the mineral illustrates the difficulties of the dispenser, and also, what is of far greater importance, the general inaccuracy of the French system. It runs thus :—

Kermes mineral	0·10 gramme
Gomme arabique	q.s.
Eau distillée	150 grammes
Teint d'aconit	6 drops
Sirop diacode	30 grammes

Frequently this would be dispensed without gum, as the quantity of powder is so small. The uncertainty as to the use of the gum is troublesome, and so is the quantity of tincture, as drop-measures are unknown. Referring to the Codex, we find that the normal drop-measure should be a glass tube with a capillary opening, having an outside diameter of 3 milli-metres, capable of giving drops of distilled water of which 20 will weigh 1 gramme. Practically these tubes are in very little use, the rough-and-ready practice of dropping from the bottle being much more prevalent—in fact, in a large dis-pensing business it would be difficult to find the time to do otherwise.

The prescription, however, has the advantage of equalling by weight exactly the contents of a 180-gramme bottle, or about an ordinary six-oz. English bottle—a circumstance for which the dispenser is always thankful. The next presents a dilemma in that respect :—

Teint d'aconit	5 drops
Teint de belladonne.	1 drop
Syrup of orange flowers	40 grammes
Eau distillée	30 ,,

In this case a 60-gramme or 2-oz. bottle will not contain the exact weight ; it has, however, been dispensed to fill both a 2-oz. and 3-oz. bottle—which makes an important difference in the dose of one teaspoonful every half-hour, and also in a 3-oz. bottle, not filled, but containing the exact weight, which an English dispenser would regard as the only correct course. But then occurs a commercial trouble. The customer complains that the bottle is not full, and that in other pharmacies this has not been the case, and he gets the impression either that he is cheated or that a mistake has been made. Moreover, it may be mentioned that French bottles are really remarkable for their inaccuracy; taking twelve bottles marked 180 grammes, perhaps one in the twelve on weighing will be found accurate, the others differing from 5 to 20 grammes.

Another example :—

Extract quinquina	1 gramme
Cognac	2 ,,
Julep gommeux	130 ,,

This mixture has been sent out both in 4-oz. and 5-oz. bottles. Many dispensers take the precaution to note the exact size of bottle in the prescription-book, so as to secure uniformity. Mixtures containing tinctures or other liquids in the quantity of 1 gramme, or even 2 grammes, are another fruitful source of discrepancies, as practically so small a dose cannot be weighed accurately into a 6 or 8 oz. bottle on an ordinary pair of counter-scales. The Codex offers some assistance with a table showing the numbers of drops contained in 1 gramme of such preparations as are most frequently prescribed; but this is not of practical service, as accurate measurement of drops involves a great loss of time. In this table the number of drops to a gramme varies from 20 of distilled water to 90 of sulphuric ether. The dispenser very soon falls into the usual system of adding these ingredients more or less 'à l'œil.'

Whilst on the subject of mixtures we note the absence in French prescriptions of a safeguard which often prevents mistakes in England. In the majority of cases French prescribers give no directions on the prescriptions as to how the medicine is to be taken. When given the directions are not infrequently shamefully vague. 'Take by spoonfuls' occurs constantly, without indication whether tea, dessert, or table spoons are intended. A consolation for the pharmacien is that French remedies are generally very innocuous, and the quantity taken is not of so much importance.

Suppositories also give rise to many uncertainties. The standard weight, according to the Codex, should be 4 grammes, which is not the case in the following :—

Cacao butter	3 grammes
Ext. opium	0·03 ,,
Ext. belladon	0·01 ,,
Camphor	0·30 ·,,

To make one suppository.

Moulds as used in England are unknown in France, and their place is roughly supplied by extemporaneous paper cones, which require some practice and dexterity to produce of the same size, so as to obtain suppositories of uniform length and diameter. It is almost certain that no two pharmacies will turn them out in identical style. Suppositories before delivery to the customer are always covered with tinfoil—for what purpose it is difficult to say, as the patient has the trouble of unwrapping each one before using.

Powders, as a rule, are dispensed in as small a compass as possible, and many pharmaciens use powder-papers already folded, with their name and address thereon. This system offers the advantage of uniformity and neatness, not always obtainable by handwork. The papers are made both in ordinary and in waxed paper, the latter being employed for iodide and bromide of sodium and other deliquescent salts, which are frequently prescribed as powders. The following is an ordinary prescription for powders :—

Calcined magnesia	0·20 gramme
Nitrate bismuth	0·20 ,,
Pancreatine	0·10 ,,
Pepsine	0·10 ,,
Prepared chalk	0·15 ,,
Opium	0·01 ,,

For one powder. Send twenty such.

The price usually charged would be *2s. 6d.* Powders are often prescribed in bulk, as the following :—

Carbonate of iron	10 g.
Peruvian bark	15 g.
Myrrh	15 g.
Liquorice	15 g.

To be taken by teaspoonfuls.

These are usually dispensed in cardboard boxes, very seldom in wide-mouth bottles, unless at the special request of the customer.

Drops offer no feature of special interest, as they do not appear to be a popular form of prescribing, and are almost confined to arsenical preparations and such tinctures as nux vomica, ignatia, &c. These are generally dispensed in stoppered bottles fitted with a capillary tube, or stoppers with a groove and lip, or, when it is a question of price, in an ordinary phial, with a separate drop tube, at a cheap rate. Collutoires, or applications for brushing out the throat or mouth, usually have as a basis mulberry syrup, honey of roses, or glycerine, with about 10 per cent. of some active ingredient, such as potassium chlorate, borax, &c. The quantity usually ordered is about 1 fluid oz., which is sent out in a wide-mouth phial sufficiently large to admit a camel's-hair brush.

The dispensing of ointments differs little from English procedure, and the formulæ do not, as a rule, present any novel features. Lard as a basis is becoming discarded for vaseline and lanolin. The preparations most in use are mercury, iodine, and zinc; turpeth mineral occurs as an ointment of 1 part in 30; also sulphate of copper. Ung. belladonnæ is a great favourite with French prescribers, and occurs in all sorts of combinations, such as the following :—

Ext. bellad.	1 g.
Ext. opii	1 g.
Ol. menth. pip.	5 gtt.
Adipis glycerinat.	20 g.

The English style of covered pots for ointments has never come into use in France, but they are usually sent out in gallipots covered with tinfoil and paper or circular discs of cardboard. Recently screw-capped jars with nickel covers have found a place on the dispensing-counter, and from their convenience and low price will soon supersede the antiquated style of package.

Syrups form the real foundation of French pharmacy. The Codex gives the formulæ of 80, all more or less in daily use, and the non-official may be reckoned at some 600, all of which occur more or less in prescriptions. Sirop de limaille de fer (syrup of iron filings) is a specimen of the more unusual ones. Here, again, discrepancies occur. The instructions of the Codex are seldom followed, as most pharmaciens prepare even the official syrups from fluid extracts. The products differ widely from the original type, especially as the admixture is frequently made out of economical motives, to avoid keeping stocks of perishable preparations. In fact, the dispensing of syrups in France is exactly parallel with that of infusions in England. It is certain, however, that this system of dispensing has told against the pharmacien; many physicians prefer to prescribe the syrups of well-known specialists—such as Laroze, Chassaing, &c.—rather than risk the home-made combinations of the dispenser. Prescriptions for specialities simply are becoming more and more common. For instance, the following :—

> One bottle digitalin (Homolle), 1 granule every two days.
> One bottle eau Gazost, as directed.
> One tin meat powder (Rousseau), a teaspoonful twice a day.
> One tube quassin (Burgraeve), one granule at each meal.

In this case nothing is left to the skill of the dispenser, and his loss of profit is very considerable. It is probable, however, that much of this has been brought about by bad work. Glucose frequently forms an important item in syrup dispensing.

Cachets, or small concave discs of wafer-paper enclosing a medicinal dose, are distinctive, and deserve to be more generally adopted. Patients like them, and they afford a good profit to the chemist. Limousin's apparatus for filling and closing the cachets is not equal to that of Digne, of Marseilles, either for simplicity or celerity. This latter is now generally adopted. An example runs :—

Pancreatin	. . . . . .	0·25 centigr.
Maltine .	. . . . . .	0·25 ,,
Bismuth .	. . . . . .	0·25 ,,
Prepared chalk	. . . . .	0·25 ,,

For one cachet. Send twenty.

The price would be 5s. Cachets are sent out in cardboard cylindrical cases of different diameters, according to size, from 0 to 3, containing from five to twenty. For the exhibition of powders, salts of quinine, &c., nothing can be better adapted than this plan, which has in many instances replaced the use of pills and powders. Cachets of quinine, bismuth, rhubarb, and other popular remedies are very generally kept ready prepared. Extracts are also prescribed in this form, as in the following formula :—

Ext. cinchonæ	. . . . .	0·15 gramme
Quininæ bromid.	. . .	0·10 ,,
Sodii salicyl.	. . . .	0·15 ,,

Make one cachet.

It is customary to mark on the prescription the size of the cachet employed, so as to secure uniformity.

Liniments are now generally dispensed in blue glass phials with distinctive red labels. The formulæ for liniments at times are very curious, as will be seen from the following :—

Tinct. digitalis.	. . . . .	15 grammes
Tinct. scillæ	. . . . .	15 ,,
Tinct. scammon.	. . . .	15 ,,
Eau de vie de lavande	. . .	300 ,,
Sulfate de quinine	. . . .	2 ,,
Ol. hyoscyami.	. . . .	200 ,,
Camphor	. . . . .	4 ,,
Laudanum (Rousseau)	. . .	4 ,,
Ext. belladon. .	. . . .	4 ,,
Chloroform	. . . . .	4 ,,

Ft. lin.

The most frequently prescribed appear to be baume opodeldoc (similar to Steer's), baume tranquille, or baume fioraventi as a basis, in conjunction with sedatives.

Pills are certainly going out of fashion, aperients being very seldom ordered in this form, nor can special pills be said to have any really popular demand. Mineral waters, such as Hunyádi Janos, Royale Hongroise, &c., have driven pills out of the field, much to the dispenser's loss. The cheap screw-capped pill tubes have superseded the old paper box, and are much adopted by specialists ; turned wood boxes appear never to have been worth making by French sundriesmen, the few met with being evidently of English origin. Some of the pill formulæ are surprising, and being frequently without any directions for taking are certainly trying to the nerves of the dispenser, *e.g.* :—

Atropinæ . . . . . 5 milligrammes
Conf. rosæ . . . . . q.s.
To make five pills.

Another :—

Veratrine . . . . . 5 centigrammes.
Opium . . . . . . 5 ,,
Ft. pil. j. Mitte xxx.

In this case, as the prescriber could not be consulted, the quantity of veratrine was changed from 5 centigrammes to $\frac{1}{2}$ centigramme.

Quassin crystal . . . . 2 milligrammes
Strychnine . . . . . $\frac{1}{2}$,,
Sulph. quinine . . . . 25 ,,
Ft. pil. j. Mitte vj.

Ext. cinchonæ . . ‹ . 10 milligrammes
Ferri lactatis . . . . . 3 ,,
Ferri et sodæ pyrophosph. . . 2 ,,
P. ergotæ . . . . . 2 ,,
Ft. pil. j. Mitte 50.

The time and care required for such preparations are never compensated by the price obtained. As a powder for rolling pills lycopodium is almost always employed, except when the pills are directed to be sent in orris or cinnamon powder, which happens occasionally. Silvering is becoming a thing of the past.

Wines are a favourite form of administration, and are usually prescribed by bottle or half-bottle; but in this case, as in so many others, proprietary articles are preferred. As examples of wines prescribed take the following :—

> Vin de quinquinæ au Malaga, containing in every 100 grammes 10 drops tinct. nucis vomicæ, send ½ litre.

or :—

> Vin. cinchonæ . . . . . . 1 litre
> Ferri et sodæ pyrophosph . . . . 2 grammes

These are usually dispensed in special-shaped bottles and capsuled.

Mélange is a word frequently employed to head the label of a preparation, and it is somewhat difficult to define, as the following specimens will show :—

I.

	grammes
Old rum	150
Creosote	5
Glycerine	20

Suivant avis (as directed).

II.

Honey	15
Extract of arnica flowers.	15

Mix.

III.

Iodoform	1
Aq. rosæ	50
Aq. destil.	50
Tinct. opii	1

Mix.

Occasionally such prescriptions as the following crop up :— Sulphate of magnesia, rose leaves, sarsaparilla, fumitory, china root, liquorice root, agaric (*Boletus laricis*), senna, and soap-wort, of each 1 oz.; infuse for twenty-four hours in 4 litres of boiling water. This involves thoroughly cutting up or disinte-

Q

grating the whole of the materials, so as to produce as uniform a compound as possible. The price charged would be 5*s*. This would be given to the patient either in a paper bag or cardboard box, according to circumstances. Packets of different preparations for infusions are frequently ordered, besides tisanes, or teas, to be drunk between the medicinal doses. Here is an example :—Quassia, 16 grammes ; roasted coffee, 32 grammes. Divide into eight packets as directed.

NEW REMEDIES.

THE present era is characterised, medicinally and pharmaceutically, by a constant stream of new medicinal agents. Some of these are commonly prescribed and present few features of difficulty in dispensing, while there are others which are rarely called for, and on that account the chemist may be unable at once to advise the physician as to how they should be administered.

In this chapter we therefore give some brief notes regarding recently introduced remedies, more especially those which are synthetically produced.

Amylene Hydrate.—This is a clear colourless liquid with a slightly camphoraceous odour; insoluble in water but soluble in alcohol and ether.

Its principal use is as a hypnotic, for which purpose the dose given is from ʒss. to ʒj.

Amylene hydrate may be administered in gelatine capsules, each containing 15 minims, or as a mixture such as the following :—

Amylen. hydrat.	ʒj.
Ext. glycyrrhiz. liq.	ʒj.
Aquæ destillat.	ad ℥j.

M. To be shaken before use.

It is sometimes administered as an enema, *per rectum*, in which case the following should be the form :—

Amylen. hydrat.	ʒj.
Mucilag. acaciæ	℥j.
Aquæ destillatæ	ad ℥ij.

Rub the amylene hydrate with the mucilage and add the water. To be shaken before use.

Anthrarobin is a synthetical product closely resembling chrysarobin, and is used as a substitute for that drug. It is found as a pale yellowish powder which is very irritating to the nostrils. It is soluble in 10 parts of glycerine at 210° C.; soluble in 10 parts of cold and 5 parts of boiling alcohol. It is insoluble in water, but is freely soluble in an aqueous solution of borax. Anthrarobin is used in place of chrysarobin in the treatment of psoriasis, herpes, and other skin diseases. It is applied in a similar way as ointment with lanolin, or in solution—alcohol, glycerine, or solution of borax being the solvent, as in the following formula:—

Anthrarobini	ʒj.
Boracis	ʒj.
Aquæ destillatæ	ʒj.

Fiat solutio.

This is the strength of preparation generally used, 1 in 5 being the strongest.

Antifebrin (Acetanilide).—This febrifuge occurs in colourless crystals, nearly insoluble in cold water, but easily soluble in alcohol. The dose is from 2 to 10 grains. Owing to the insolubility of antifebrin in water it is not easy to give it in mixture form, because that necessitates a large proportion of alcohol. The following is a good form :—

Antifebrin	ʒj.
Syrupi	ʒj.
Spt. vini Gallici	ad ℥vi.

Dissolve the antifebrin in the brandy and add the syrup. ℥ss. is the common dose of this mixture for an adult.

Antifebrin is, however, best given in pill form—glycerine of tragacanth is the excipient to use—in compressed tablets, or in powders with wafer-paper.

Antipyrin, originally introduced as a febrifuge, but also extensively used as a soporific and for other purposes, occurs in colourless laminar crystals, which dissolve both in alcohol and water very readily. The doses vary from 15 to 30 grains for an adult, and from 3 to 12 grains for children. Five grains make a good though large pill with 1 grain of tragacanth powder and a tiny drop of water.

The hypodermic injection is made according to the following formula :—

Antipyrin	ʒj.
Aquæ destillat.	ʒij.

Dissolve by the aid of heat.

A good whooping-cough mixture for children is made as ollows :—

Antipyrin	gr. xv.
Vin. Tokay	ʒj.
Aquæ destillat.	ʒj.
Syr. flor. aurantii	ʒj.

Fiat mistura.

Dose. A tablespoonful every two hours.

When prescribed as powders it is preferable to dispense the crystalline form of antipyrin. The remedy is also largely given in the form of compressed tablets.

Antithermin.—This is one of the latest synthetical bodies recommended as febrifuges. It occurs in crystalline form, the substance is colourless, insoluble in water, and difficultly soluble in alcohol. No account has yet been given of its therapeutic action or posology. It can be administered as powders or pills, like antifebrin.

Aseptol (Sozolic Acid).—A syrupy-like fluid of a reddish colour, soluble in water, alcohol, and glycerine. Used externally as an antiseptic. Aseptol must not be mistaken for the aseptinic acid of commerce. It is generally dispensed in aqueous solution—1 part of aseptol to 20 to 30 parts of water—and should be sent out in blue glass bottles.

Betol—a remedy for rheumatism—occurs in brilliant crystals, insoluble in water, but soluble in alcohol and fixed oils. Dose, 15 to 30 grains in powder or pills. Betol bougies

(weight 20 grains, each containing 4 grains of betol) are made
with cacao-butter.

Bromethyl (Bromide of Ethyl).—A colourless, volatile
fluid possessing an odour like chloroform. Its specific gravity
should be 1·390 if pure. It is used as an anæsthetic, like chloroform. Care should be taken to keep and dispense the fluid
in distinctive bottles, so that it may not be mistaken for other
fluids, more especially for *bromethylene*, which has quite different
properties.

Creolin.—Jeye's Disinfectant is sold in Germany under
this name. The chemical-like name has something probably
to do with its success. It is administered internally in doses
of 2 to 5 minims in catarrh of the bladder; is used externally
as an ointment (5 to 10 minims to 1 ounce); and as an injection
in gonorrhœa (5 to 25 minims to 1 ounce).

Guaiacol—one of the principal constituents of creosote—
is a colourless liquid, soluble in ether, alcohol, and fixed oils,
but only sparingly soluble in water. It is used as a remedy
in phthisis, in doses of a minim three times a day, given in
mixture, or along with cod-liver oil. Thus:—

Guaiacol.	℥ xv.
Spirit. rectificat.	℥i.
Aquæ destillatæ	℥viij.

M.

Dose. A tablespoonful in a glassful of water twice a day.

Guaiacol	℥ x.
Ol. morrhuæ	℥v.

Misce.

Hydrargyri Carbolas.—This new salt of mercury has
been introduced as the safest mercuric salt for administration
in syphilis. It is in the form of colourless crystalline needles,
nearly insoluble in water, and difficultly soluble in alcohol.
Dose, $\frac{1}{3}$ to $\frac{1}{2}$ grain. It is the mercuric, not the mercurous, salt
which should be used, and pills are the best form for adminis-
tration. The following formula is recommended :—

Hydrargyri carbolat.. . . . . . gr. 20
Pulv. glycyrrhizæ . . . . . . ʒj.
Ext. glycyrrhizæ . . . . . . ʒj.

Fiat massa, et divide in pilulas sexaginta. To be coated with tolu.

Hydrargyri Salicylas.—An amorphous white powder, difficultly soluble in water and alcohol, easily soluble in an aqueous solution of sodium chloride or sodium bicarbonate. Used in the treatment of syphilis, gonorrhœa, and similar diseases. Internally given in doses not exceeding 1 grain daily, in syphilis, and used as an injection for gonorrhœa. The following are suitable forms for dispensing the remedy:—

Pills.

Hydrargyri salicylatis . . . . . gr. xv.
Pulv. glycyrrhizæ . . . . . . ʒj.
Extracti glycyrrhizæ . . . . . ʒj.

Misce, fiat massa et divide in pilulas sexaginta (60).

Injection.

Hydrargyri salicylatis . . . . . gr. j.
Sodii bicarbonatis . . . . . . gr. xv.
Aquæ destillatæ . . . . . . ʒv.

Fiat solutio.

To be used four or five times a day.

Hypnone is a colourless fluid, sparingly soluble in water, and more soluble in alcohol. Dose, 3 to 8 minims as a hypnotic.

Hypnone exerts a somewhat caustic action upon the mucous membrane, and for that reason it is best dispensed in gelatine capsules, each of which should contain 1 minim of hypnone dissolved in 9 minims of almond-oil.

Ichthyol (Ammonium Ichthyolate).—A dark-brown and thickish fluid, insoluble in water, but soluble in alcohol and ether. Internally ichthyol is given in doses of 4 to 20 minims, but it is much more used externally as an ointment with lanolin, and in other forms. For this purpose the ammonium ichthyolate is generally used, but it is preferable to use the sodium ichthyolate for pills, as that salt is much thicker than the ammonium one. A good solution of ichthyol for spray is made by dissolving one part of ammonium ichthyolate in two parts of spirit of ether.

Iodine Terchloride.—A yellowish-red substance, which is very hygroscopic and is therefore kept in sealed glass tubes. Its principal use is as an antiseptic. It is also useful as an anti-fermentative in dyspepsia, and as an injection in gonorrhœa. Iodine terchloride is supplied in 15-grain tubes, sufficient to make 4 ounces of lotion (about 1 per ·cent.). It forms a mahogany-coloured solution with water, which must be protected from the action of light, as this converts it into a mono-chloride, which, however, has also antiseptic power. This change is rapidly effected on coming in contact with organic matter, chlorine and iodine being liberated in a nascent state. Hence the action as an antiseptic.

Iodol.—A pale yellowish-brown powder used as a substitute for iodoform. It is insoluble in water, but soluble in alcohol and fixed oils. For the same purposes as iodide of potassium it is given internally in doses of 1 to 2 grains, dispensed in pill form. Thus:—

Iodol	gr. xii.
Pulv. glycyrrhiz.	gr. xii.
Ext. glycyrrhiz.	gr. xii.

Fiat massa, et divide in pilulas xii.

Externally it is used, like iodoform, chiefly as a dusting powder, but also in the form of ointment.

Kairin.—A febrifuge which enjoyed considerable reputation for some time, but is not now manufactured, antipyrin having taken its place.

Methylal.—A colourless ethereal fluid, readily soluble in water, alcohol, and fixed oils. Dose as a hypnotic, 15 to 30 minims. Is also used externally as a local anæsthetic, being applied in the form of ointment or liniment (with oil), both of which should, owing to the extremely volatile nature of methylal, be dispensed in well-stoppered bottles.

A good mixture for internal use :—

Methylal	. ʒij.
Syr. flor. aurantii	. ʒi
Aquæ destillatæ	ad ℥ij.

Dose, a tablespoonful.

Mollin.—This is an oleo-saponaceous ointment basis which does not melt even in the warmest climate. It is white, and of the consistency of lard. The great advantage of it is that it can be easily washed off the skin, whether it is used in the pure state or mixed with such medicaments as Peruvian balsam, ichthyol, and the like. In dispensing ointments containing mollin, the medicaments, if soluble, may first be dissolved before incorporating with the base, or the dry substance and the mollin may be intimately mixed in a mortar.

Morrhuol is a proprietary article, which is represented to be the active principle of cod-liver oil.

Naphthalin is found in the form of colourless crystals which possess an odour like coal-gas. The substance is insoluble in water, sparingly soluble in cold alcohol and fixed oils, and readily soluble if heated with these solvents.

Therapeutically, naphthalin is used internally in the treatment of typhoid fever (2 to 8 grains), and externally in skin diseases. It is also used for the preservation of natural history specimens from the attack of moths and other small insects. Owing to the insoluble nature of the drug, it should not be given in the form of mixture, but as powders. The following formula is a good one, as it ensures that the disagreeable odour of the naphthalin is disguised :—

Naphthalini	. gr. xxx.
Sacchari albi	. gr. xxx.
Olei bergamotti	. ♏j.

Misce et divide in pulveres duodecim.

A powder may be given three times a day.

In preparing ointments of naphthalin the drug should be dissolved in the melted fatty basis.

Naphthol occurs in resplendent crystalline scales, nearly insoluble in cold water, but very soluble in alcohol and fixed oils. It is used externally as ointment or in alcoholic solution in the treatment of skin diseases, scabies, &c. The ointment is made by dissolving the naphthol in the melted fatty basis, the general strength varying from 1 in 20 to 1 in 10. For itch the stronger preparation is most beneficial. The solution (1 in 40) is simply used as an antiseptic wash for the skin.

Oxynaphthoic Acid.—There are two modifications of this body, viz., the *alpha* and *beta*, but it is the former which is used as an antiseptic. It is a nearly white powder, practically insoluble in water, but soluble on the addition of alkalies, which form salts with it. The acid is easily soluble in alcohol and ether. In addition to its properties as an antiseptic, oxynaphthoic acid is also used as an antizymotic. At present, however, itch appears to be the only complaint for which the acid has come into use, and for this purpose a 1 in 20 ointment (with lanolin or vaseline), or, better, a collodion containing 2 grains per ounce, is beneficial.

Paraldehyd.—This modification of aldehyd is not now so much used as it was, but, like other new remedies which have not fulfilled all that was anticipated of them, it is occasionally prescribed. It is a colourless liquid, soluble in 10 parts of water, and soluble in alcohol. Dose, ʒss. to ʒj. as a hypnotic. The following makes a good sleeping draught :—

Paraldehyd .	ʒj.
Spiritus vini gallici	ʒss.
Olei limonis .	♏j.
Syrupi .	ʒss.
Aquæ .	ad ℥iij.

M.

Phenacetin (Paracetphenetidin).—This, one of the latest of the synthetical compounds introduced as antipyretics, is a white crystalline powder, nearly insoluble in water, but easily soluble in alcohol. It is perfectly tasteless. The dose of it is from 8 to 20 grains for adults as an antipyretic, and similar doses may be given in neuralgia, for which phenacetin also appears to be useful. It is best given in powder form or as tablets, its insoluble character not permitting it to be made into mixture.

Photoxylin.—This is collodion made from wood-wool gun-cotton. It has practically the same applications as the official collodion.

Pyridine.—Used for inhalation in asthma. It is a colourless fluid, soluble in water and alcohol. A fluid drachm of it is used for each inhalation, being simply poured upon a plate and inhaled.

Resorcin occurs in colourless crystals, readily soluble in water and alcohol. It is used internally in doses of 8 to 20 grains as an antifermentative and antipyretic, and externally in the form of ointment or solution in the treatment of skin diseases and in urethral affections. The following is a suitable form for an injection :—

Resorcin	30 grs.
Aq. destill.	℥iv.
Solve.	

Saccharin.—A white powder, sometimes possessing a weak odour of bitter almonds owing to impurity, very slightly soluble in water, but soluble in alcohol. With alkalies it forms salts which are freely soluble in water. Saccharin possesses an extraordinarily sweet taste, and is also slightly antiseptic. It is solely used for its sweetening properties, and in mixtures is preferably combined with a little bicarbonate of soda. Acids, of course, throw it out of solution.

Salol.—A white crystalline powder, insoluble in water, but soluble in alcohol. Combines the properties of phenol and salicylic acid (of which it is a compound), and, like the latter, is used in the treatment of acute rheumatism, and also as an antiseptic, like iodoform. It is much used as a mouth-wash and gargle for correcting foetid breath. The dose of salol is from 15 to 30 grains three times a day, dispensed as powders.

Salufer, the proprietary name of fluosilicate of soda solution. Mr. Wm. Thomson, of Manchester, has found the fluosilicates to be powerfully antiseptic. Fluosilicate of soda is soluble in about 180 parts of water, and the solution salufer (a patented article) is used in 2 per cent. mixture with water as an antiseptic lotion in surgical operations; also as an injection in gonorrhœa, and as a gargle in diphtheria.

Solvin (Polysolve).—A yellowish, oily liquid, soluble in 2 parts of water, but the substance is thrown out of solution on the addition of more water. It mixes freely with alcohol, ether, chloroform, turpentine, and glycerine. It dissolves such substances as sulphur, iodoform, naphthalin, salicylic acid, salol, chrysarobin, camphor, asafœtida, cantharidin, and santonin to the extent of 1 in 50. It is owing to this latter property that it is used in medicine as a basis for liniments and ointments. It should be kept in perfectly full bottles, as it becomes thick on exposure to the air.

Sozoiodol.—The substance found in commerce under this name is a soda salt of iodparaphenolsulphonic acid. Various other salts are also to be had, and they are more or less soluble in water. All are white crystalline solids.

Sozoiodol is an iodoform substitute, used externally as an ointment, or the powder is sprinkled on the affected parts. The following is a good recipe for the ointment:—

Sozoiodol	.	.	.	.	.	.	ℨij.
Zinci oxidi	.	.	.	.	.	.	℥ss.
Amyli	.	.	.	.	.	.	ℨj.
Vaselini	.	.	.	.	.	.	℥iss.

Fiat unguentum.

Lanolin may be used in place of vaseline.

Sulphonal—the latest hypnotic—is in the form of white crystals, which dissolve in about 12 parts of boiling water, but the substance is much less soluble in cold water, one ounce dissolving a grain with difficulty. Alcohol and ether dissolve it more readily. Dose: 15 to 30 grains five hours before bedtime.

In addition to being practically insoluble in cold water sulphonal does not mix well with it, and requires a little mucilage of acacia for its suspension, or the following may be used :—

Sulphonal	ʒss.
Pulv. tragacanthæ comp.	gr. vj.
Syrupi	ʒij.
Aquæ	ad ℥iss.

Rub the sulphonal in a mortar to fine powder, add the compound tragacanth powder, mix, then add the water and syrup to form a uniform mixture.

If it is desired to give sulphonal in solid form, the compressed tablets should be ordered, as pills are comparatively bulky, owing to the quantity of excipient required.

Terpine Hydrate.—A colourless crystalline solid, difficultly soluble in cold, but more soluble in hot, water, and soluble in alcohol. Used in bronchitis and other chest affections. Dose: 3 to 10 grains. The following are suitable forms for administration :—

Pills.

Terpin. hydrat.	ʒj.
Glycerin. tragacanth.	q.s.
Fiat massa. Divide in pilulas xxx.	

Mixture.

Terpin. hydrat.	ʒj.
Glycerini	℥ij.
Spirit. rectificat.	℥ij.
Syrupi	℥ij.

Mix the terpine hydrate with the glycerine, heat on a water-bath until dissolved, and add the spirit and syrup previously mixed.

Terpinol is a colourless, oily liquid, insoluble in water, but soluble in alcohol and ether. Its uses are the same as terpin hydrate. Dose: 2 grains. It is best given in gelatine capsules, the dose being mixed with three times its volume of olive oil. It may also be given in pills, such as :—

Terpinol	ʒj.
Ammonii benzoatis	ʒj.
Ceræ flavæ	ʒj.
Acaciæ pulveris	gr. xx.
Sacchari albi	gr. xx.
Pulv. glycyrrhizæ	gr. xx.
Mucil. tragacanthæ	q.s.

Fiant pilulæ xl.

Thallin.—Since the introduction of antipyrin and phenacetin, thallin has not been so much asked for. The sulphate of the base is generally used. It is a crystalline, colourless solid, soluble in water and less soluble in alcohol. Internally it is given in doses of 3 to 8 grains made into pills. For gonorrhœa it is used as an injection, 4 to 8 grains in an ounce of water, and as bougies with the cacao-butter basis.

Tribromophenol is used medicinally as an antiseptic. It is a solid in very soft white crystals, scarcely soluble in water, but soluble in alcohol. For surgical dressings the powder is simply sprinkled on cotton wool and applied to the part, or an ointment containing 10 grains or more to the ounce of vaseline is used. The dose internally is 1 to 2 grains.

Urethan (Ethyl Carbamide) is a white crystalline solid, soluble in water and alcohol. Used as a hypnotic in doses of 15 to 40 grains, given in powder or tabloids, or as a draught. For the latter the following is suitable :—

Urethan	ʒij.
Syrupi	ʒj.
Aquæ	ad ʒiv.

M.

Dose: Two tablespoonfuls.

HOMŒOPATHIC DISPENSING.

HOMŒOPATHIC DISPENSING is one of the simplest matters in the world, and therefore requires but very little description. In prescriptions, medicines are ordered in the form of mixtures or powders, and never contain more than one active ingredient.

To those not familiar with homœopathic prescriptions, a few examples will best serve to explain their mystery :—

I.

Trit. sulphur (3)   .   .   .   .   .   .   gr. j.
Ft. pulvis. Mitte x. Sumat unam in aquæ coch. una; om. nocte h.s.

To dispense the above 10 grains of sulphur trituration (3) are to be mixed with about 30 grains of sugar of milk, and the whole divided into ten powders. Great care should always be observed in the outer manipulation of homœopathic prescriptions, and, indeed, this remark applies to all dispensing The powders are usually covered separately with tinfoil, in order to preserve their properties.

II.

Aconiti nap. glob.   .   .   .   .   .   . $^2/_3$
Sacch. lactis q.s., ft. pulvis, una quartis horis super linguam capienda. Mitte xx.

In this case globules are to be used—two in each powder. Unless specially stated, 3 grains of sugar of milk is the proportion for each powder. It will be noted that the difference in the directions given is, that in the first instance the dose is to be dissolved, while in the second it is taken dry on the tongue.

III.

Tinct. nucis vomicæ	$^{12}/_6$
Aquæ destill.	℥vj.

M. Ft. mistura, cujus capiat cochlearia duo magna tertiis horis.

In the last two instances the figures following the medicine indicate the number of drops or globules, and the attenuation. In the third, for example, *twelve* drops of the *sixth* dilution are prescribed for the mixture.

IV.

Nucis vomicæ . . . $^2/_3$ Belladonnæ . . . $^2/_5$
Sacch. lactis. . . . q.s.   Sacch. lactis . . . q.s.

    Ft. pulvis. Mitte vj. Sign. 1, 3, 5, 7, 9, 11.   Ft. pulvis. Mitte vj. Sign. 2, 4, 6, 8, 10, 12.

One powder to be taken alternately, in the order they are numbered, every two hours.

V.

Merc. vivi . . . . $^2/_3$ Sacch. lactis . . . gr. iij.
Sacch. lactis . . . q.s.   Ft. pulvis. Mitte iij. Sign 4, 5, 6.

    Ft. pulvis. Mitte iij. Sign. 1, 2, 3.

The powders are to be taken every four hours in the order they are numbered.

The above prescriptions (Nos. 4, 5) are specimens of homœopathic prescriptions in the first of which it is desired to give nux vomica and belladonna in alternation. In the next case it is evident that the object is for the patient to take no medicine during the second day.

In prescribing pilules and globules some practitioners write their directions as follows :—

Pil. chamomillæ . . . . . . $^3/_{12}$

Direct a pilule to be taken every three hours.

Glob. belladonnæ . . . . . . $^6/_6$
Sacch. lactis . . . . . . q.s.

Ft. pulv. Direct to be dissolved in three tablespoonfuls of water, and tablespoonful to be taken every six hours.

In the first of these prescriptions 12 pilules of chamomilla are ordered. These would, of course, be dispensed in a bottle. In the second six globules of belladonna 6 are to be rubbed down with about 30 grains of sugar of milk. In both cases the centesimal dilutions are intended.

The indication of the quantity and the attenuation, as shown in the two articles, varies. Some prescribers write $^3/_{12}$ and some $^{12}/_3$ for 12 drops of the third dilution. The dispenser must judge from the prescription and from his knowledge of the prescriber's usual practice.

The following specimens of the various forms of homœopathic prescribing have been written by an eminent homœopathic physician. They comprise all varieties of prescriptions likely to be met with from English homœopathic practitioners, and a very few words will suffice to make clear any possible difficulties which might present themselves to a dispenser not previously familiar with such prescriptions.

It is not necessary to give facsimile specimens, as the average caligraphy of the homœopathic prescribers is above that of their allopathic rivals, and directions are always written in English.

The Greek θ indicates the matrix, or mother, tincture, and the number immediately following the name of the medicine ordered indicates the dilution. If an x be added, the decimal scale of dilution is intended ; in all other cases the centesimal scale is understood.

MIXTURES.

Tinct. nucis vom. 3x.   .   .   .   .   ♏ xij.
Aquæ destill. .   .   .   .   .   .   ℥iij.

Ft. m.   Direct a dessertspoonful to be taken every six hours.

Tinct. bryoniæ alb. θ .   .   .   .   ♏ xij.
Aquæ dest.   .   .   .   .   .   ℥iij.

Ft. m.   Direct a dessertspoonful to be taken every three hours.

R

POWDERS.

It is usual to wrap each powder separately in tinfoil over the white paper.

> Trit. mercurii sol. 3x. . . . . . gr. $\frac{1}{2}$

Mitte tales chart, xij. Direct a powder to be taken dry on the tongue every four hours.

> Tinct. pulsat. 6 . . . . . . ♏ vj
> Sacch. lactis . . . . q.s.

Ft. pulv. Direct this powder to be dissolved in six tablespoonfuls of water, and a tablespoonful to be taken every morning and evening.

> Glob. ignatiæ 6 . . . . . . iij.
> Sacch. lactis . . . . q.s.

Ft. pulv. Mitte tales, xij. Direct a powder to be taken every four hours.

PILULES.

> Pil. sulph. 12. . . . . . . xxiv.

Direct two pilules to be taken every morning and evening.

APPLICATIONS.

> Tinct. arnicæ θ . . . . . . ℥ss.
> Aquæ destill. . . . . . . ℥viij.

Ft. lotio.

Label.—For external application.

Direct a piece of lint in three folds to be soaked in the lotion, applied to the bruise, and covered with oiled silk.

> Linim. rhus . . . . ℥ij.
> Linim. saponis simplicis. . . . . ℥iv.

Ft. linimentum.

Label.—For external application.

Direct to be gently rubbed into the joint every four hours.

ILLEGIBLE PRESCRIPTIONS.

THE capability of pharmacists to decipher illegible caligraphy is so generally known as to be almost proverbial. It is a kind of expertness which they have acquired through long practice in reading the prescriptions of physicians. Their business requires this art; it has received official recognition by being made a part of the requirements of the qualifying examination, at which badly-written medical prescriptions have to be read by candidates, and teachers find it necessary to collect specimens of bad medical penmanship on behalf of their pupils.

The duty of the dispenser who has an illegible prescription presented to him has never been clearly defined; he has certainly a perfect right, legally, to refuse to compound a prescription which he cannot read; but it is believed that in the case of prescriptions which have previously been dispensed he is justified in doing his best. The best, however, may be a serious matter to the patient if it happens to be contrary to the intentions of the prescriber. It is far better for the dispenser that he should not risk his own reputation or the comfort of his customer by undertaking a task respecting which he is uncertain.

We subjoin a few examples of such prescriptions which have actually been dispensed. The study of these may afford assistance to any who have had little practice in deciphering obscure caligraphy. It is important to remember that in deciphering handwriting the peculiarities of the specimen should be picked out. These frequently give a clue to the whole thing, and once a writer's style has been grasped, difficulties in the future appear to vanish. This is the case with the following :—

The above is a prescription of Dr. Cecil W. Hastings, 'a well-known bad writer,' remarked a correspondent of *The Chemist and Druggist* at the time the facsimile was first published. The most difficult point about it is the quantity of the second ingredient of the 'drops'; opinions are divided as to whether it should be ♏ v or ℥ss. The former is, however, on the whole more in accordance with the writer's style, for, in the case of the other drachm signs, they are distinctly separated from the names of the ingredients, whereas the opposite is the case with the 'ol. menth. pip.' The translation is :—

℞ Benzole . . . . ℥ij.
Ol. menth. pip. . . . . . . ♏v.
Ol. olivæ . . . . ℥x.

F. mist. Cap. gutt. xxx. t. die.

C. W. H.

℞ Calomel . . . . g. iv.
Pulv. Doveri . . . . ℥ij.
Bism. subnit. . . . . . . ℈ij.
Ol. carui . . . . q.s.

Misce. Ft. pil. xxiv. Cap. j. 2 horis.

C. W. H.

The next specimen is much less obscure :—

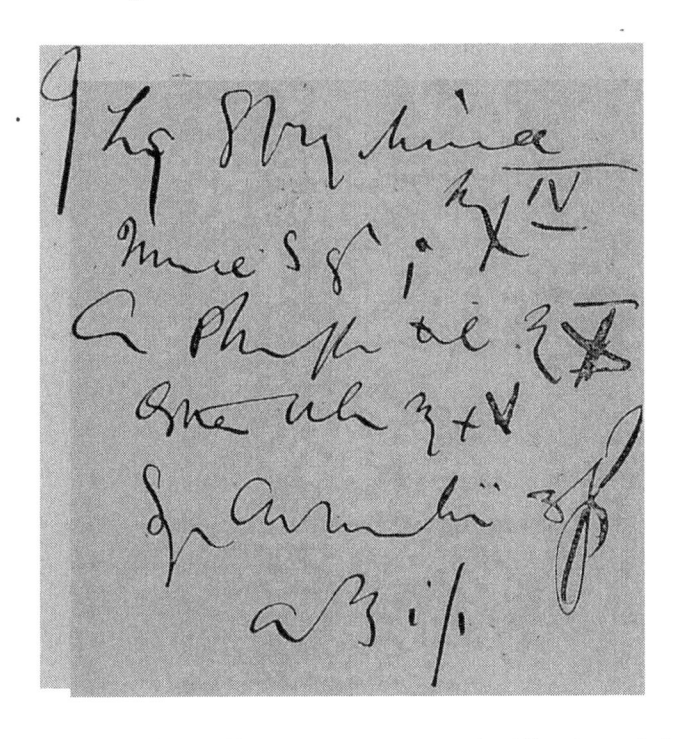

The quantity of liquor strychniæ looks like ' ♏ xiv,' but this is not intended. Dr. Ward Cousin is the writer of this, and the rendering is :—

℞   Liq. strychniæ   . . : . . . . ℥ iv.
      Quin. s. .   . . . gr. j.
      Ac. phosph. dil. .   . . . ℥ x.
      Æther. chlor. .   .   .   .   .   . ℥ xv.
      Syr. aurantii   .   .   .   .   .   . ℥ss.
      Aq.   .   .   .   . ad ℥iss.

The subjoined prescription is an extremely carelessly written one, of the 'scrap of paper' class which cause numerous mistakes :—

The peculiarity of this prescription lies in the contraction 'y' for 'every.' The proper rendering is :—

℞   Disulph. quinæ   .   .   .   .   .   . ℥ss.
      Bromid. sodii .   .   .   :   .   . ℥ij.
Divid. in pulv. xij.

One y 8hrs.

℞   Liq. ferri chloroxidi.   .   .   .   .   . ℥j.
20 drops in water y [8 hours].

The words in parentheses are written along the left-hand side
A most misleading prescription is the following :—

No less than eight different renderings of this have been given by experienced dispensers. It was rendered as follows by the pharmacist who sent it to *The Chemist and Druggist* :—

Haust. ferri aper. bis.

Alum   .   .   .   . ʒiv.

ʒij. ad Oss aquam (*sic*) once day.

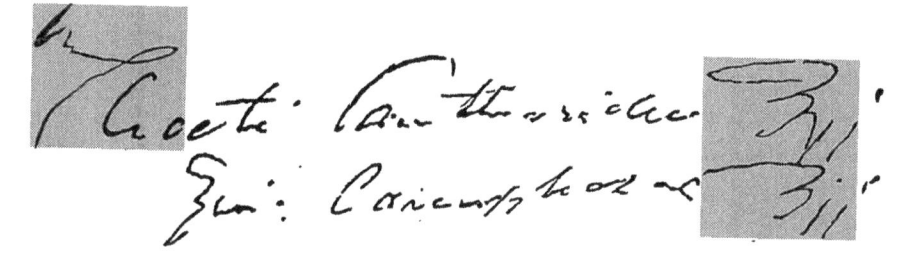

This last is a carelessly written prescription, the second ingredient being particularly obscure ; but after careful examination the dispenser will render it :—

℞   Aceti cantharidis   .   .   .   .   . ʒvj.

   Spir. camphoræ   .   .   .   .   . ʒij.

This is correct. There is little in the writing to guide the dispenser, but it is highly unlikely that the writer would mean 'Lin. camphoræ' (an oleaceous preparation) to be mixed with a vinegar.

EXAMINATION PRESCRIPTIONS.

THOSE who use this volume preparatory to entering for the qualifying examination will find the following prescriptions useful for practice. They have been given by the Boards in Edinburgh and London during the past three years, and are not likely to be given again. We do not comment upon these prescriptions, so far as giving the best method of procedure, the object of printing them here being to make them exercises for students. Four to six articles are generally given to each candidate, but in some cases more may be given, and the whole have to be dispensed within two hours.

Tr. ferri perchlorid.   .   ℨij.
Potass. tart. .   .   ℨj.
Aquæ . . .   ad ℨvj.
  M. Ft. mist. ℨss. bis die.

Atropiæ sulph.   . .   gr. $\frac{1}{24}$
Ol. theobrom.   . .   q.s.
  Ft. suppos. Mitte vj.

———

Ext. belladon.   . .   gr. iij.
Ol. theobrom.   . .   q.s.
  Ft. suppos. Mitte vj. .

Hyd. perchlor.   . .   gr. ij.
Ext. coloc. co.   . .   gr. iij.
  Ft. pil. Mitte xij., quarum cap.
  unam om. noct. si opus sit.

Bals. copaibæ . .   ℥ss.
Pul. gum. acac. . .   ℨij.
Liq. potassæ .   . .   ℨj. .
Tinct. opii . .   Ʒij.
Sp. æther. nit.   .   ℨiij.
Aq. . . . . ad ℥iv.
  Capt. ℨss. q.q. quart. horâ.

———

Tr. cannab. ind. . .   ℨij.
Tr. card. co. .   .   ℨiij.
Aq. . . .   ad ℥iv.
  M. Ft. mist. sec. art. Coch.
  mag. j. t. d. s.

Pulv. opii . . .   gr. iij.
Potass. nit. .   . .   gr. xv.
  M. Ft. pulv. tres. j. bis die
  sum.

Potassii iodid.	gr. xxx.
Potassii carb.	gr. x.
Adipis .	ad ℥j.

M. Ft. ung. m. d. utend.

Ammon. carb.	℈j.
Tr. tolu	ʒij.
Tr. camph. co.	ʒij.
Pulv. tragac. co.	gr. viij.
Aquæ .	ad ℥iv.

M. Ft. mist. Coch. mag. ter quaterve die sum.

Ferri sulph.	gr. iss.
Pil. aloes et myrrh.	gr. iv.

M. Ft. pil. Mitte xij. Una t. d. sumend.

Phosphori	gr. $\frac{1}{30}$
Ferri redact.	gr. iij.

M. Ft. pil. Mitte xxiv.

Emp. canthar. pone sinistram aurem ponendam.

Mag. sulph.	℥j.
Mag. carb.	℥ss.
Tr. lavand. co.	ʒij.
Pot. iodid.	ʒss.
Tr. aurantii	℥ss.
Aq. menth.	ad ℥viij.

M. Ft. mist. Cujus æger cap. coch. unum ter in die in cyatho vinario aq. frig. post jentac., prand. et cœn.

Ol. ricini	ʒiij.
Ol. terebinth.	ʒij.
Gum. acaciæ.	ʒij.
Aq.	ad ℥iv.

M. Ft. mist. Cap. ℥ss. q.q. quartâ sextâve horâ.

Plumbi acet.	gr. xiv.
Pulv. opii	gr. xx.
Adipis .	℥ss.

Ft. ung. m. d. s.

Acet. plumbi	gr. iij.
Pulv. opii	gr. j.
Ol. theobrom.	q.s.

Ft. suppos. Mitte vj.

Ferri sulph.	gr j.
Ext. hæmatoxyli	gr. ij.
Ext. hyoscyami	gr. j.

M. Ft. pil. Mitte xij. j. t. d.

'Send a piece of white leather spread with emp. plumbi 8 by 2 inches.'

Aq.	ad ℥vj
Ol. amygd.	ʒvj.
Liq. potass.	ʒvj.
Liq. morph., P.B.	ʒiss.

M. ℥ss. ter quaterve die.

('Send ½ quantity of mixture.')

Pulv. rhei	gr. ij.
Creosoti	♏ j.
Sapo.	gr. j.

M. Ft. pil. Mitte octo. Cap. j. ter die dum opus sit (post cibos).

P. cret. aromat.	ʒj.
Rhei	gr. xl.
Mucil. tragac.	℥j.
Aquæ .	ad ℥iv.

M. Ft. mist. Capiat 4tam part. pro dosi s, o, s.

Potass. chlor. . . . gr. xl.
Tinct. tolutan. . . . ℨij.
Glycerin. . . . ℨij.
Syrup. simp. . . ℨij.
Aquæ . . . ad ℥iv.
    Mis. Ft. garg. subind utend.

Hyd. chlor. . . . gr. xij.
    M. Ft. pil. x. Cap. j. c. sing.
    dos. m. seq.

———

Plumbi acet. . . gr. xxx.
Opii . . . . gr. iij.
    M. Ft. pil. [xii.] One every
    night.

Pulv. rhei . . . ℨss.
Sodæ bicarb. . . ℨj.
Bismuthi carb. . . ℨij.

Mucil. trag. . . . ℥iij.
Sp. amm. co. . . ℨj.
Aq. . . . . ad ℥vj.
    M. Fiat mist. C. coch. j. mag.
    quâ quâ horâ et coch. ij. h.s.s.

———

Hyd. c. cretâ . . gr. iij.
Pulv. rhei . . . gr. viij.
    Misce tere in pulverem. Capiat
    quamprimum mane.

Liq. ammon. fort. . ℨij.
Ol. amygd. . . . ℨiv.
Camphoræ . . . ℨj.
Chlorof. . . . ℨij.
Tinct. opii . . . ℨiss.
Aquæ . . . ad ℥ij.
    Misce. Part. dolent. applicand.

The above represent twelve sets of articles, to be dispensed in as many hours.

APPENDIX

—◆◆—

TERMS LIKELY TO OCCUR IN FRENCH AND GERMAN PRESCRIPTIONS.

A, *Fr.*, to, or; Trois à quatre paquets (three or four powders).

Abendessen, Abend -brod, -mahlzeit, -tisch, *Ger.*, supper. Drei von diesen Pillen vor dem Abendessen. (Three of these pills before supper.)

Acide azotique, *Fr.*, nitric acid.

Aetz, *Ger.*, caustic.

Aetzstein, *Ger.*, caustic potash.

Alcohol sulphuris, *Ger. Lat.*, carbon bisulphide.

Alcohol de soufre, *Fr.*, carbon bisulphide.

Altschädenwasser, *Ger.*, lotio flava, yellow wash.

Aqua calcaria, *G.L.*, lime water.

Aqua chlorata, *G.L.*, chlorine water.

Arsenige Säure, *Ger.*, arsenious acid.

Arsensäure, *Ger.*, arsenic acid.

Augenstein, *Ger.*, lapis divinus.

Azotate, *Fr.*, nitrate.

Barbotine, *Fr.*, santonica.

Baudruche, *Fr.*, goldbeater's skin.

Bisse, *Ger.*, bolus. Sechs Bissen im Tage zu nehmen auf drei Gaben vertheilt. (Six boluses to be taken daily, divided into three doses.)

Blauholz, *Ger.*, logwood.

Bleiessig, *Ger.*, liq. plumbi subacet.

Bol, *Fr.*, bolus. A prendre six bols par jour en les partageant en trois doses. (Six boluses to be taken every day, dividing them into three doses.)

Bourdaine, *Fr.*, rhamnus frangula.

Calcaria, *G.L.*, calx or calcium.

Carboneum, *G.L.*, carbon.

Carbonicum, *G.L.*, carbonas, or carbonate.

Cautère potentiel, *Fr.*, caustic potash.

Chamomilla vulgaris, *G.L.*; Matricaria chamomilla, *L.*

Chaux, *Fr.*, lime.

Chinin, *Ger.*, quinine.

Chininum, *G.L.*, quinine.

Chloratum, *G.L.*, chloride.

Chlorsaures, *Ger.*, chlorate.

Cinchonium, *G.L.*, cinchonine.

Citricum, *G.L.*, citrate.

Coccionella, *G.L.*, cochineal.

Colla piscium, *G.L.*, icthyocolla.

Coton cardé, *Fr.*, wadding, cotton wool.

Coucher, *Fr.*, bed-time, going to bed. A prendre deux pilules avant le coucheur. (Two pills to be taken at bed-time.)

Cyanatum, *G.L.*, cyanidum, cyanide.

Cuillerée à café, *Fr.*, teaspoonful. Une cuillerée à café au cas d'une attaque de toux. (A teaspoonful to be taken if the cough comes on.)

Cuillerée à soupe, *Fr.*, tablespoonful. Prenez une cuillerée à soupe toutes les deux heures. (One tablespoonful every two hours.)

Dower'sche Pulver, *Ger.*, Dover's powder.

Eau de Rabel, *Fr.*, mixtura sulphurica acida.

L'Effet voulu, *Fr.*, the desired effect. Une cuillerée à café toutes les demi-heures jusqu' à l'effet voulu. (A teaspoonful every half-hour till it acts.)

Einspritzung, *Ger.*, injection.

Eisessig, *Ger.*, glacial acetic acid.

Emplastrum adhæsivum anglicum, *G.L.*, court plaster.

Emplastrum picatum, *G.L.*, pitch plaster.

Essen, *Ger.*, meals,

Essig, *Ger.*, vinegar.

Esslöffel, *Ger.*, tablespoon. Alle zwei Stunden einen Esslöffel voll. (A tablespoonful every two hours.)

Ferrocyanatum, *G.L.*, ferrocyanide.

Flasche, *Ger.*, bottle. Schütteln Sie die Flasche. (Shake the bottle well.)

Fois, *Fr.*, time. Prenez en quatre fois à une demi-heure d'intervalle. (To be taken in four portions at intervals of half an hour.)

Gouttes, *Fr.*, drops. A prendre dix gouttes trois fois par jour. (Ten drops to be taken thrice daily.)

Glas, *Ger.*, glass, tumbler.

Hirschtalg, *Ger.*, mutton suet.

Höllenstein, *Ger.*, silver nitrate, lunar caustic.

Iodure de formyle, *Fr.*, iodoform.

Kohlensäure, *Ger.*, carbonic acid.

Kümmel, *Ger.*, caraway.

(A) Jeun, *Fr.*, fasting. Prenez deux ou trois de ces pilules à jeun. (Take two or three of these pills fasting.)

Latwerge, *Ger.*, electuary.

Lavement, *Fr.*, enema.

Limonade sèche, *Fr.*, effervescent saline.

Liqueur de belloste, *Fr.*, liquor hydrargyri nitratis acidus.

Liquiritia, *G.L.*, glycyrrhiza.

Mal, *Ger.*, time, portion. Auf vier Mal in halbstündigen Zwischenräumen zu nehmen. (To be taken in four portions at intervals of half an hour.)

Malva arborea, *G.L.*, althæa rosea, *L.*, hollyhock.

Mittagsessen, *Ger.*, dinner (properly

' mid-day meal '). Dieses Pulver unmittelbar vor dem Mittagsessen zu nehmen. (This powder to be taken immediately before dinner.)

Natrium, *G.L.*, sodium ; Natrum, *G.L.*, soda, sodium oxide.

Nüchtern, *Ger.*, sober, fasting. Vier oder sechs von diesen Pillen nüchtern zu nehmen. (Four or six of these pills to be taken fasting, or before breakfast.)

Oblate, *Ger.*, wafer. Ein Pulver vor der Mahlzeit in einer Oblate zu nehmen. (A powder to be taken in a wafer before meals.)

Ordonnance, *Fr.*, prescription.

Ouate, *Fr.*, wadding, cotton wool.

Pain azyme, *Fr.*, wafer. Un de ces paquets à prendre dans du pain azyme avant le repas. (One of these powders to be taken in a wafer before meals.)

Paquet, *Fr.*, a packet, powder. A prendre un paquet toutes les deux heures. (One powder to be taken every two hours.) On prend un de ces paquets peu de temps avant l'attaque de fièvre. (One of these powders to be taken shortly before the fever fit.)

Pasta gummosa, *G.L.*, pâte de guimauve.

Pastilles, *Fr.*, lozenges. A prendre de quatre à six pastilles par jour. (Four to six lozenges to be taken daily.)

Pastillen, *Ger.*, lozenges. Man nimmt von diesen Pastillen auf einmal nur eine alle zwei Stunden. (One only of these lozenges to be taken every two hours.)

Paullinia, *Ger.*, guarana. ..

Pierre à cautère, *Fr.*, caustic potash.

Pillen, *Ger.*, pills. Zwei Pillen jeden Abend vor dem Zubettegehen. (Two pills every evening at bed-time.)

Pilules, *Fr.*, pills. Deux pilules chaque soir avant le coucher. (Two pills every evening at bed-time.)

Pincée, *Fr.*, a pinch. Infusez une pincée de ces herbes avec un demi-litre d'eau bouillante pour faire un tisane. (Infuse a pinch of these herbs in half a pint of water to make a draught.)

Potasse à la chaux, *Fr.*, caustic potash.

Potion, *Fr.*, mixture, potion.

Poudre, *Fr.*, powder. Matin et soir une poudre dix minutes avant le repas. (One powder every morning ten minutes before meals.)

Poudre alexitère, *Fr.*, pulv. ipecac. co.

Poudre anodine, *Fr.*, pulv. ipecac. co.

Poudre diaphoretique, *Fr.*, pulv. ipecac. co.

Poudre gazeuse ou gazifere purgative, *Fr.*, seidlitz powder.

Poudre gazogene, *Fr.*, effervescent or gazogene powder.

Poudre gazogene neutre, *Fr.*, soda powder.

Poudre gazogene laxative, *Fr.*, seidlitz powder.

Poudre Savory, *Fr.*, seidlitz powder.

Poudre sudorifique, *Fr.*, pulv. ipecac. co.

Priser par le nez, *Fr.*, to snuff. Pour priser par le nez cinq ou six fois par jour. (To be snuffed five or six times daily.)

Pulver, *Ger.*, powder. Ein Pulver jeden Morgen und Abend zehn Minuten vor dem Essen. (One powder every morning and evening ten minutes before meals.) Man nimmt ein Pulver kurz vor dem Fieberanfall. (A powder to be taken shortly before the fever fit.)

Pulvis aërophorus, *G.L.*, effervescent powder, gazogene powder, soda powder.

Pulvis aërophorus laxans, *G.L.*, seidlitz powder.

Pulvis gummosa, *G.L.*, pulvis tragacanthæ co.

Räucherkerzchen, *Ger.*, fumigating pastilles.

Räucheressig, toilet or disinfecting vinegar.

Remède du capucin, *Fr.*, liquor hydrargyri nitratis acidus.

Remède du duc d'Antin, *Fr.*, liquor hydrargyri nitratis acidus.

Repas, *Fr.*, meals.

Rezept, *Ger.*, prescription.

Rhodomel, *Fr.*, mel rosæ.

Riechessig, *Ger.*, aromatic vinegar.

Saindoux, *Fr.*, lard.

Säure, *Ger.*, acid.

Schlafengehen, *Ger.*, bed-time. Vor dem Schlafengehen zwei Pillen zu nehmen. (Two pills to be taken at bed-time.)

Schnupfen, *Ger.*, to snuff. Fünf bis sechs Mal im Tage zu schnupfen. (To be snuffed five or six times daily.)

Schwarzeswasser, *Ger.*, black wash, lotio nigra.

Schwefel, *Ger.*, sulphur.

Schwefligesäure, *Ger.*, sulphurous acid.

Schwefelsäure, *Ger.*, sulphuric acid.

Sebum, *G.L.*, sevum, suet.

Sel de lait, *Fr.*, milk sugar.

Semen cine, *Fr.*, santonica.

Soufre végétal, *Fr.*, lycopodium.

Stibium, *G.L.*, antimonium.

Sucre de Saturne, *Fr.*, lead acetate.

Sulfuratum, *G.L.*, sulphidum, sulphuretum, sulphide.

Sulfuricum, *G.L.*, sulphas, sulphate.

Table, *Fr.*, table. Se mettre à table. (To dine.) A prendre deux de ces pilules en se mettant à table. (Two pills to be taken before dining.)

Taffetas d'Angleterre, *Fr.*, court plaster.

Tartarus boraxatus, *G.L.*, soluble tartar, potassium boro-tartrate.

Tartarus depuratus, *G.L.*, potassium acid tartrate, cream of tartar.

Tartarus natronatus, *G.L.*, Rochelle salt, sodium potassium tartrate.

Tartarus stibiatus, *G.L.*, emetic tartar, antimonium tartaratum.

Theelöffel, *Ger.*, teaspoon. Ein Theelöffelvoll, a teaspoonful.

Tisane, *Fr.*, draught, medicated drink.

Tische, *Ger.*, table. Zu Tische gehen. (To dine.) Man nehme zwei von diesen Pillen wenn man zu Tische geht. (Take two pills before dining.)

Trifolium fibrinum, *G.L.*, Menyanthes trifoliata, buckbean.

Tropfen, *Ger.*, drop. Drei Mal des Tages zehn Tropfen zu nehmen. (Ten drops to be taken thrice daily.)

Verordnung, *Ger.*, prescription.

Verre, *Fr.*, glass, tumbler. Un verre d'eau sucrée. (A tumbler of sugar and water.) .

Wasserstoff, *Ger.*, hydrogen.

Weinsteinsäure, *Ger.*, tartaric acid.

Wirkung, *Ger.*, action, effects. Ein Theelöffelvoll alle halbe Stunden bis zur Wirkung zu nehmen. (Take a teaspoonful every half-hour till it acts.)

Zahnwurzel, *Ger.*, pellitory root.

Zeste, *Fr.*, the peel of oranges, lemons, &c.

Zittwersamen, *Ger.*, santonica.

Zubettegehen, *Ger.*, bed-time.

Zuckersäure, *Ger.*, oxalic acid.

ABBREVIATIONS USED IN PRESCRIPTIONS.

A., (1) *aa, ana*, of each ingredient ; (2) *ab, absque* ; of or from ; (3) *adde*, add thou ; (4) *ante*, before ; (5) *alternus*, alternate ; (6) *aqua*, water ; (7) *artem, secundum artem*, according to art ; (8) *asinus, lac asini*, asses' milk.

A. H., *alternis horis*, every other hour.

A. J., *ante jentaculum*, fasting, or before breakfast.

A. P., *ante prandium*, before dinner.

Abdom. *abdomen*, the abdomen, the belly.

Abs. febr., *absente febre*, fever being absent.

Acid. hydroc., (1) *acidum hydrochloricum* ; (2) *acidum hydrocyanicum*.

Aconit., (1) *aconitum*, the plant ; (2) *aconitina*, aconitine.

Ad 2 vic., (1) *ad secundam vicem*, to the second time ; (2) *ad duas vices*, for two times.

Ad 3tiam vicem, *ad tertiam vicem*, for three times.

Ad def. animi, *ad defectionem animi*, to fainting.

Ad del. animi, *ad deliquium animi*, to fainting.

Ad gr. acid., *ad gratam aciditatem*, to an agreeable acidity.

Ad libit., *ad libitum*, at pleasure.

Ad recid. præc., *ad recidivum præcavendum*, to prevent a relapse.

Add., (1) *adde*, add thou ; (2) *addantur*, let them be added ; (3) *addendus*, to be added ; (4) *addendo*, by adding.

Adeps S., *adeps suillus*, hog's lard.

Adjac., *adjacens*, adjacent.

Admov., (1) *admove*, apply ; (2) *admoveatur*, let it be applied ; (3) *admoveantur*, let them be applied.

Ads. febre, *adstante febre*, while the fever is present.

Adv., *adversum*, against.

Æger, Ægra, the patient or sick.

Aggred. febre, *aggrediente febre*, while the fever is coming on.

Alter. (altern.) horis, *alternis horis*, every other hour.

Alvo adst., *alvo adstricta*, when the bowels are confined.

Ammon, (1) *ammonia* ; (2) *ammoniacum*.

Aq. astr., *aqua astricta*, frozen water.

Aq. bull., *aqua bulliens*, boiling water.

Aq. com., *aqua communis*, common water.

Aq. dest., *aqua destillata*, distilled water.

Aq. ferv., *aqua fervens*, warm, or hot, water.

Aq. fluv., *aqua fluviatilis*, river water.

Aq. font., *aqua fontana*, vel *fontis*, vel *fontalis*, spring water. (Has been misread, aqua *fortis*.)

Aq. gel., *aqua gelida*, cold water.

Aq. mar., *aqua marina*, sea water.

Aq. niv., *aqua nivalis*, snow water.

Aq. pluv., *aqua pluviatilis*, seu *pluvialis*, rain water.

Auris, the ear.

B., (1) *balsamum*, a balsam; (2) *balneum*, a bath; (3) *bene*, well; (4) *bis*, twice; (5) *bolus*, bolus, a large pill; (6) *bovis* (lac b., *lac bovis*, cow's milk); (7) *brachium*, the arm (mitt sang. b., *mittatur sanguis brachio*, let blood be taken from the arm); (8) *bulliens*, boiling.

Bb., bbds., *barbadensis*, Barbadoes.

B.M., *balneum maris* seu *marinum*, a sea or salt water bath.

B.P., B.Ph., British Pharmacopœia.

B.T., *balneum tepidum*, a warm bath.

B.V., *balneum vaporis, vaporosum*, a vapour bath.

Bib. *bibe*, drink thou.

Bis ind., *bis indies*, twice a day.

Brachium, the arm.

Bull., (1) *bulliens*, boiling; (2) *bulliat* or *bulliant*, let boil.

But., *butyrum*, butter.

C. (1) lac c., *lac capellæ, lac capræ*, goat's milk; (2) c. radat., *caput radatur*, let the head be shaved; (3) p.c. *post cænâm*, after supper, *pondus civile*, avoirdupois; (4) *colatus*, strained; (5) *coletur*, let it be strained; (6) *compositus*, compound; (7) *concisus*, cut or bruised; (8) *confectio*, a confection; (9) *congius*, a gallon; (10) *conserva*, a conserve; (11) *continua*, continue thou; (12) *contritus*, bruised, broken small; (13) *contusus*, bruised, pounded; (14) *cortex*, bark; (15) *crastinus*, of to-morrow; (16) *crystalis*, in crystals; (17) *cujus*, of which; (18) *cum*, with; (19), *cyathus*, a glass pot or cup.

C.C., (1) *cucurbitula cruenta*, a cupping-glass with a scarificator; (2) *cornu cervi*, hartshorn.

C.C.U., *cornu cervi ustum*, burnt hartshorn.

C.M.S., *cras mane sumendus*, to be taken to-morrow morning.

C.N., *cras nocte*, to-morrow night.

C. radat, *caput radatur*, let the head be shaved.

C.V., *cras vespere*, to-morrow evening.

C. theæ, *cyatho- theæ*, in a cup of tea.

C. vinar., *cyathus vinarius*, a wine-glass.

Cærul., *cæruleus*, blue.

Cal. calom, *calomelas*, calomel; (2) *calidus*, warm.

Calc. chlor., (1) *calcii chloridum*, calcium chloride; (2) *calcis chloratæ*, of chlorinated lime.

Cap., *capiat*, let (the patient) take.

Caput r., *caput radatur*, let the head be shaved.

Cataplasma, a poultice.

Charta, a paper (a powder in paper).

Co., *compositus*, compound.

Coch., *cochleare, cochlearium*, spoonful.

Coch. ampl., *cochleare amplum*, a large (table) spoonful; about 4 fl. drachms.

Coch. inf., *cochleare infantis*, a child's spoonful.

Coch. mag., *cochleare magnum*, a large or table spoonful, about 4 fl. drachms.

Coch. med. *vel* mod., *cochleare medium* vel *modicum*, a middling (dessert) spoonful, about 2 fl. drachms.

Coch. parv., *cochleare parvum*, a small (tea) spoonful; about 1 fl. drachm.

Cochleat., *cochleatim*, by spoonfuls.

Col., (1) *cola*, strain; (2) *colatus*, strained.

Colat., (1) *colatus*, strained; (2) *colaturæ*, to the strained liquor; (3) *colatur*, let it be strained.

Colet., *coletur*, let it be strained.

Colent., *colentur*, let them be strained.

Color., *coloretur*, let it be coloured.

Comp., *compositus*, compound.

Con., *concisus*, cut, sliced.

Cong., *congius*, a gallon.

Cons., *conserva*, (1) a conserve; (2) keep thou.

Cont. rem. *seu* med., *continuentur remedia* seu *medicamenta*, let the medicines be continued.

Coq., (1) *coque*, boil; (2) *coquentur*, let them be boiled.

Coq. ad med. consumpt., *coque* seu *coquetur ad medietatis consump-* *tionem*, boil, or let it be boiled, till half is consumed.

Coq. s. a., *coque secundum artem*, boil according to art.

Coque in s. a., *coque in sufficiente quantitate aquæ*, boil in a sufficient quantity of water.

Cort., *cortex*, bark.

Crast., *crastinus*, for to-morrow.

Crus, the leg.

Cuj., *cujus*, of which.

Cujusl., *cujuslibet*, of any.

Cyath. theæ, *cyatho theæ*, in a cup of tea.

Cyath., *cyathus, vel* c. vinar., *c. vinarius*, a wineglass; about 2 fluid ounces, or in France about 5 fluid ounces.

D., (1) d. sp., *debita spissitudo*, a proper consistence; (2) *detur*, let it be given; (3) *dexter*, the right side; (4) *dies*, a day; (5) *dilutus*, diluted; (6) *dimidium*, the half; (7) *directio*, a direction; (8) *divide, dividatur*, divide thou, let it be divided; (9) *donec*, until; (10) *dosis*, a dose; (11) *dum*, until; (12) *duplex*, double; (13) *durans*, during; (14) *duratus*, dried.

D. in 2plo, *detur in duplo*, let twice as much be given.

D. in p. æq., *dividatur in partes æquales*, let it be divided into equal parts.

D. P., *directione propriâ*, with a proper direction.

D. spiss., *debita spissitudo*, a proper consistence.

Deaur. pil., *deaurentur pilulæ*, let the pills be gilded.

De d. in d., *de die in diem*, from day to day.

Deb. spiss., *see* D. spiss.

Dec., *decanta*, pour off.

Decub., *decubitûs,* of lying down.

Decub. hor., *decubitûs horâ,* at the hour of going to bed, at bed-time.

Deglut., *deglutiatur*, let it be swallowed.

Dej. alvi, *dejectiones alvi*, stools.

Det., *detur*, let it be given.

Dext. lat., *dextrum latus*, the right side.

Dieb. alt., *diebus alternis*, every other day.

Dieb. tert., *diebus tertiis*, every third day.

Dil., (1) *dilue*, dilute thou; (2) *dilutus*, diluted.

Diluc., *diluculo*, at break of day.

Dim., *dimidius,* one-half.

Donec alv. bis dej., *donec alvus bis dejiciatur*, until the bowels have been twice evacuated.

Donec alv. sol. fuer., *donec alvus soluta fuerit*, until the bowels be opened.

Donec dol. neph. exulav., *donec dolor nephriticus exulaverit*, until the nephritic pain is removed.

E., (1) *electus*, picked or selected; (2) *electuarium*, an electuary; (3) *emeticum*, an emetic; (4) *emplastrum*, a plaster; (5) *eos*, the morning; (6) *extractum*, an extract; (also as a preposition—of, out of).

Eburn., *eburneus*, made of ivory.

Ed., *edulcorata*, edulcorated, clarified.

Ejusd., *ejusdem*, of the same.

Elect., *electuarium*, an electuary.

Emp. lyth., *emplastrum lythargyri*. (Has been misread emplastrum lyttæ.)

Enem., *enema*, an enema, a clyster.

Ex gel. vit., *ex gelatinâ vituli*, in calves'-foot jelly.

Exhib., *exhibeatur*, let it be exhibited.

Ext. col., (1) *extractum colchici* ; (2) *extractum colocynthidis*.

Ext. sup. alut. moll., *extende super alutam mollem*, spread it upon soft leather.

F., (1) *fac*, make thou; (2) *fiat, fiant*, let it (them) be made; (3) *fervens*, boiling; (4) *folium*, a leaf; (5) *forma*, form, shape; (6) *fortis*, strong; (7) *fotus*, a fomentation; (8) *fuscus*, brown.

F.H., *fiat haustus*, let a draught be made.

F.L.A., *fiat lege artis*, let it be made by the rules of art.

F.M., *fiat mistura*, let a mixture be made.

F.S.A., *fiat secundum artem,* let it be made according to art.

F. pil., (1) *fac pilulas*, make pills; (2) *fiant pilulæ*, let pills be made.

F. venæs, *fiat venæsectio*, bleed.

Facies, the face.

Fasc., *fasciculus*, a bundle which can be carried under the arm; about 4 oz. *Linnæus*, 1 oz. *Geiger*.

Feb. dur., *febre durante*, during the fever.

Fem. intern., *femoribus internibus*, to the inner part of the thighs.

Fict., *fictilis*, earthen.

Fil., *filtrum*, a filter.

Fist. arm., *fistula armata*, a clyster pipe and bladder fitted for use.

Fl., (1) *flatus*, flatulence; (2) *flavus*, yellow; (3) *flos*, a flower; (4) *fluidus*, fluid, or by measure;

(5) *fluviatilis,* aq. fl., river water.

Fol., *folium,* leaf.

Frust., *frustillatim,* in little pieces.

Ft., *fiat, fiant,* let it be made.

G., (1) *gallicus,* French; (2) *gelatina,* jelly; (3) *gelida,* aq. g., cold water; (4) *gummi,* a gum; (5) *granum,* a grain; (6) *gutta,* a drop.

G.G.G., *gummi guttæ gambæ,* gamboge.

Gargarisma, a gargle.

Gel. quav., *gelatina quavis,* in any kind of jelly

Genu, knee.

Gr., *granum,* a grain.

Gr. vj. pond. *grana sex pondere,* six grains by weight.

Gtt., *gutta,* a drop; *guttæ,* drops.

Gutt. quibusd., *guttis quibusdam,* with a few drops.

Guttat., *guttatim,* by drops.

H., (1) *habeat,* he may have, let him have; (2) *horum,* of these; (3) *haustus,* a draught; (4) *herba,* a herb; (5) *hic,* this; (6) *hora,* an hour; (7) *hujus,* of this.

H.D., *horâ decubitûs,* at bed-time, at the hour of going to bed.

H. p. n., *haustus purgans noster,* our purging draught (made by a private formula).

H.S., *horâ somni,* at the hour of sleep.

Har. pil. sum. iij., *harum pilularum sumantur tres,* let three of these pills be taken.

Hb., *herba,* a herb.

Hirudo, a leech.

Hor. iima. mat., *horâ undecimâ matutinâ,* at 11 A.M., at the eleventh hour in the morning.

Hor. interm., *horis intermediis,* in the intermediate hours.

Hor. un. spat., *horæ unius spatio,* at the expiration of an hour.

Hydr., (1) *hydrargyrum,* mercury; (2) *hydras,* hydrate; (3) *hydriodas,* iodide; (4) *hydrochloricum,* hydrochloric; (5) *hydrocyanicum,* hydrocyanic.

Hydr. bic., (1) *hydrargyri bichloridum,* corrosive sublimate; (2) *hydrargyri bicyanidum,* bicyanide of mercury.

Hydr. bin., (1) *hydrargyri biniodidum,* biniodide of mercury; (2) *hydrargyri binoxidum,* red oxide of mercury.

Hydr. chlor., (1) *hydrargyri chloridum,* calomel generally, (strictly corrosive sublimate); (2) *hydras chloral,* chloral hydrate.

Hydr. ox. n., (1) *hydrargyri oxidum nigrum,* black oxide of mercury; (2) *hydrargyri oxidum nitricum,* red oxide of mercury.

Ignis, fire.

In pulm., *in pulmento,* in gruel.

Inc., *incide,* cut thou; (2) *incisus,* cut, sliced.

Ind., *indies,* from day to day, daily.

Inf., *infunde,* pour in; (2) *infricare,* to rub in; (3) *infusum,* an infusion.

Inj. enem., *injiciatur enema,* let an enema or clyster be (thrown up) administered.

J., *jentaculum,* breakfast.

Jul., *julepus, julepum, julapum,* a julep.

Kal. ppt., *kali præparatum,* prepared kali, potassium carbonate.

L., (1) *lac,* milk; (2) *lapis,* a stone; (3) *latus,* a side; (4) *lege,* (¹) read thou, (:) by law; (5) *libra*, a pound, also a pair of scales; (6) *lignum*, wood; (7) *linimentum*, a liniment; (8) *liquor*, a liquor or liquid; (9) *lotio*, a lotion.

Lac A., *lac asinarum*, asses' milk.

Lac B., *lac bovis*, cow's milk.

Lac C., *lac capræ* seu *capellæ*, goat's milk.

Lac O., *lac ovillum* seu *ovinum*, ewe's milk.

Lac V., *lac vaccæ*, cow's milk.

Lat dol., *lateri dolenti*, to the painful or affected side.

Lenis, gentle.

M., (1) *mane*, the morning; (2) *manipulus*, a handful; (3) *marina*, marine, belonging to the sea; (4) b.m., *balneum maris*, a sea-water bath; (5) *massa*, a mass; (6) *mensurâ*, by measure; (7) m. pan., *mica panis*, crumb of bread; (8) *minimum*, a minim; (9) *misce*, mix thou; (10) *mitte*, send; (11) *mistura*, a mixture.

M.B., *misce bene*, mix well.

M.P., *massa pilularum*, a pill mass.

M. dict., *more dicto*, in the way directed.

Menth. p., (1) *mentha piperita*, peppermint; (2) *mentha pulegium*, pennyroyal.

M. pan., *mica panis*, crumb of bread.

Man., *manipulus*, a handful.

Mane pr., *mane primo*, very early in the morning.

Min., (1) *minimum*, a minim; (2) *minutum*, a minute.

Mic. pan., *mica panis*, crumb of bread.

Mitt., (1) *mitte*, send; (2) *mittatur*, *mittantur*, let it, let them, be sent.

Mitt. sang. ad ℥xij. saltem, *mitte sanguinem ad uncias duodecim saltem*, take blood to 12 oz. at least

Mod. præsc., *modo præscripto*, in the manner prescribed.

Mor. dict., *more dicto*, in the manner directed.

Mor. sol., *more solito*, in the usual manner.

Mr., *mistura*, a mixture.

N., (1) *natura*, nature; (2) *niger*, black; (3) *nocte*, at night; (4) *nomen*, name; (5) *non*, not; (6) *novus*, new; (7) *nucha*, *nucha capitis*, the nape of the neck; (8) *numero*, in number; (9) *nux*, a nut.

N.M. *nux moschata*, nutmeg.

N. capit, *nucha capitis*, the nape of the neck.

Ne tr. s. num., *ne tradas sine nummo*, do not deliver unless paid.

Ng., *niger*, black.

Nisi, unless.

No., *numero*, in number.

O., (1) *octarius*, a pint; (2) *oleum*, oil; (3) *omnis*, all; (4) *optimus*, the best; (5) *ovillum* and *ovium*, sheep's, belonging to sheep; (6) *ovum*, an egg.

Oculus, the eye.

O.M., *omne mane*, every morning

O.N., *omne nocte*, every night.

O.O.O., *oleum olivæ optimum*, best olive oil.

O. alt. hor, *omnibus alternis horis*, every alternate hour.

Ol. lini s. i., *oleum lini sine igne*, cold-drawn linseed oil.

Omn. bid., *omni biduo*, every two days.

Omn. bih., *omni bihorio*, every two hours.

Omn. hor., *omni horâ*, every hour.

Omn. man., *omne mane*, every morning.

Omn. noct., *omni nocte*, every night.

Omn. quadr. hor., *omni quadrante horæ*, every quarter of an hour.

Ov., *ovum*, an egg.

Oz., the ounce avoirdupois, as distinguished from the troy or apothecaries' ounce (written ℥).

P., (1) *pars*, a part ; (2) *parvus*, small ; (3) *per*, by ; (4) *pilula*, a pill ; (5) *pilus*, hair ; (6) *pondere*, by weight ; (7) *pondus*, weight ; (8) *præparatus*, prepared ; (9) *prandium*, dinner ; (10) *pro*, for ; (11) *proprius*, proper ; (12) *pulvis*, a powder.

P. æ., *partes æquales*, equal parts.

P. c., *pondus civile*, civil weight, avoidupois weight.

P. d., *per deliquium*, by deliquescence.

P. m. (1) *pondus medicinale*, medicinal weight, apothecaries' weight ; (2) *post meridiem*, the afternoon.

P. r. n., *pro re natâ*, occasionally.

P. derad., *pilus deradatur*, let the hair be shaved off.

P. rat. æt., *pro ratione ætatis*, according to the age of the patient.

Part. aff., *partem affectam*, the part affected.

Part. dolen., *partem dolentem*, the part in pain.

Part. vic., *partitis vicibus*, in divided doses.

Past., *pastillus*, a lozenge, pastille.

Pectus, the breast, chest.

Per. op. emet., *peractâ operatione emetici*, when the operation of the emetic is finished.

Per salt., *per saltum*, by leaps (speaking of blood from an artery).

Ph. B., *Pharmacopæia Britannica*, British Pharmacopœia.

Ph. D., *Pharmacopæia Dublinensis*, Dublin Pharmacopœia.

Ph. E., *Pharmacopæia Edinensis*, Edinburgh Pharmacopœia.

Ph. L., *Pharmacopæia Londinensis*, London Pharmacopœia.

Ph. U.S., United States Pharmacopœia.

Plen. riv., *pleno rivo*, in a full stream.

Pocil., *pocillum*, a little cup.

Pocul., *poculum*, a cup ; a tea-cup holds 4 to 6 fl. oz.

Post sing. sed. liq., *post singulas sedes liquidas*, after every liquid stool.

Potass. hydr., *see* Hydr. potass.

Ppt., *præparata*, prepared.

Pr., mane pr., *mane primo*, very early in the morning.

Prandium, dinner.

Pro pot. com., *pro potu communi*, for a common drink.

Prox. luc., *proximâ luce*, on the next day.

Pug., *pugillus*, a pinch.

Pulv., (1) *pulvis*, a powder ; (2) *pulverisatus*, powdered.

Pv., *parvus*, small.

Q., (1) *quantum*, as much ; (2) *quisque, quaque*, &c., everyone ; (3) *quorum*, of which ; (4) *quaterve*, or four times ; (5) *quatuor*, four ; (6) *qui*, who, which, any ; (7) *quorum*, of which.

Q. *l.*, *quantum libet*, as much as you please.

Q. p., *quantum placet*, as much as you please.

Q. q. h., *quaque quartâ hora*, every four hours.

Q. s., *quantum satis* seu *sufficiat*, as much as is sufficient.

Q. v., *quantum vis*, vel *volueris*, as much as you will.

Quor., *quorum*, of which.

R., (1) caput r., *caput radatur*, let the head be shaved ; (2) *radix*, a root ; (3) p. r. n., *pro re natâ*, occasionally ; (4) *recipe*, take thou ; (5) *rectificatus*, rectified ; (6) *redactus*, reduced or powdered ; (7) *regio*, region, part.

R. in pulv., red. in pulv., *redactus in pulverem*, powdered.

Redig. in pulv., *redigatur in pulverem*, let it be reduced to powder.

Reg. hep., *regio hepatis*, the region of the liver.

Reg. umbil., *regio umbilici*, the umbilical region.

Repet., *repetatur*, *repetantur*, let it (them) be repeated.

S., (1) *sal*, a salt ; (2) *semina*, seeds ; (3) *semis*, half ; (4) *si*, if ; (5) *simul*, together ; (6) *sine*, without ; (7) *sit*, *si opus sit*, if there be occasion ; (8) *spiritus*, spirit ; (9) *stratum*, a layer ; (10) *succus*, juice ; (11) *adeps s.*, *adeps suillus*, hog's lard ; (12) *sufficiens*, sufficient ; (13) *sumo*, *sumere*, to take ; (14) *super*, upon ; (15) *syrupus*, syrup.

S. a., *secundum artem*, according to art.

S. G., specific gravity.

S. N., *secundum naturam*, according to nature.

S. o. s., *si opus sit*, if there be occasion.

S. S. S., *stratum super stratum*, layer upon layer.

S. s., *semis*, seu *semissis*, half.

S. v., (1) *spiritus vini*, spirit of wine ; (2) *spiritus vinosus*, ardent spirits of any sort.

S. v. m., *spiritus vini methylatus*, methylated spirit.

S. v. r., *spiritus vini rectificatus*, rectified spirit.

S. v. t., *spiritus vini tenuior*, proof spirit.

Scat., *scatula*, a box.

Scrob. cord., *scrobiculus cordis*, the pit of the stomach.

Semidr., *semidrachma*, half a drachm.

Semih., *semihora*, half an hour.

Seq. luce, *sequenti luce*, the following day.

Sesunc., *sesuncia*, an ounce and a half.

Sesquih., *sesquihora*, an hour and a half.

Si. n. val., *si non valeat*, if it does not answer.

Si op. sit, *si opus sit*, if there be occasion.

Si vir. perm., *si vires permittant*, if the strength permitt.

Signat., *signatura*, a label.

Sig. n. pr., *signetur nomine proprio*, let it be written upon or signed with the proper, and not the trade, name.

Sing., *singulorum*, of each.

Sod. chlor., (1) *sodii chloridum* ; (2) *soda chlorata* or *chlorinata*, chlorinated soda.

Ss., *semis, semissis*, half.

St., *stet, stent*, let it (them) stand.

Sternum, the breast-bone, chest.

Sub fin. coct., *sub finem coctionis*, when the boiling is nearly finished.

Sulph., (1) *sulphur*; (2) *sulphas*, a sulphate; (3) *sulphidum, sulphuretum*, a sulphide.

Sum., (1) *summitates*, the summits or tops; (2) *sume*, take thou; (3) *sumat*, let him take; (4) *sumatur*, let it be taken; (5) *sumantur*, let them be taken; (6) *sumendus*, to be taken.

Sum. tal., *sumat talem*, let the patient take one like this.

T., (1) *talis*, such as, like this; (2) *tenuis*, thin, weak; (3) *tere*, rub (thou); (4) *tinctura*, a tincture.

T.O., *tinctura opii*, tincture of opium.

T.O.C., *tinctura opii camphorata*, camphorated tincture of opium, paregoric elixir.

T. s., *tere simul*, rub together.

Tabel., *tabella*, a lozenge.

Temp. dext., *tempori dextro*, to the right temple.

Tr., Tra., *tinctura*, a tincture.

Trit., *tritura*, triturate.

Troc., *trochisci*, lozenges.

Ult. præscrip., *ultimo præscriptus*, the last ordered.

Usq. ut liq. anim., *usque ut liquerit animus*, until fainting is produced.

U.S.Ph., United States Pharmacopœia.

V., (1) *venæ*, the veins; (2) *vesper*, the evening; (3) *vinum*, wine; (4) *vis. quantum vis*, as much as you will; (5) *vitellus*, yolk (of eggs); (6) *vitulus*, a calf; (7) *volueris, quantum volueris*, as much as you wish.

V.O.S., *vitello ovi solutus*, dissolved in yolk of egg.

Vom. urg., *vomitione urgente*, the vomiting being troublesome.

V. s., *venæsectio*, bleeding, vene section.

Vices, times.

Zz., *zingiber*, ginger.

A TABLE SHOWING THE USUAL INTERNAL DOSES FOR ADULTS OF THE MORE ACTIVE MEDICINAL AGENTS, ARRANGED ALPHABETICALLY.

The prefix B.P. indicates that the substance is contained in the British Pharmacopœia of 1885. The asterisk * that, although contained in the B.P., the dose is not given and has been taken from other sources.

Solids by Weight ; Fluids by Measure	Grains or Minims		Solids by Weight ; Fluids by Measure	Grains or Minims	
B.P. Acidum arseniosum	$\frac{1}{60}$ to $\frac{1}{12}$		B.P. Calcii hypophosphis	5	10
B.P. ,, carbolic. cryst.	1	3	B.P. ,, chloridum	3	10
B.P. ,, hydrobrom. dil.	15	50	B.P. ,, sulphidum	$\frac{1}{10}$	1
B.P. ,, hydrocyan. dilut.	2	8	B.P. Cambogia	1	4
,, ,, Scheele	1	2	B.P. Camphora	1	10
B.P. ,, phosph. conc.	2	5	Cannabin tannate	2	10
B.P. Aconitina *	$\frac{1}{240}$	$\frac{1}{60}$	B.P. Cantharis *	$\frac{1}{2}$	1
B.P. Æther	20	60	Capsicin	$\frac{1}{4}$	$\frac{1}{2}$
B.P. ,, acetic	20	60	B.P. Capsici fructus *	$\frac{1}{2}$	1
Agaricin	$\frac{1}{12}$	$\frac{1}{6}$	B.P. Chloral hydras	5	30
B.P. Aloïnum	$\frac{1}{2}$	2	Chlorodyne	5	10
Ammon. arsenias	$\frac{1}{10}$	$\frac{1}{2}$	B.P. Chloroformum	3	10
B.P. Amyl. nitris (vapour)	2	5	B.P. Chrysarobinum	$\frac{1}{8}$	$\frac{1}{2}$
B.P. ,, ,, by mouth	$\frac{1}{2}$	1	B.P. Cocainæ hydrochlor.	$\frac{1}{4}$	1
B.P. Antimonii oxidum	1	4	B.P. Codeïna	$\frac{1}{4}$	2
B.P. ,, sulphurat.	1	5	B.P. Colchici cormus	2	8
B.P. ,, tart. (emetic)	1	2	Colchicinum	$\frac{1}{30}$	—
B.P. ,, ,, (diaphoret.)	$\frac{1}{16}$	$\frac{1}{4}$	B.P. Colocynthidis pulpa	2	8
Antipyrin	5	30	B.P. Confectio opii	5	20
B.P. Apomorphinæ hydrochlor. * (by mouth)	$\frac{1}{16}$	$\frac{1}{4}$	B.P. ,, scammonii	10	30
B.P. Apomorphinæ hydrochlor. * (hypoderm.)	$\frac{1}{24}$	$\frac{1}{8}$	B.P. Conii folia	2	8
B.P. Aqua laurocerasi	30	120	Conina	$\frac{1}{4}$	—
B.P. Argenti nitras	$\frac{1}{4}$	$\frac{1}{3}$	Convallamarin	$\frac{1}{2}$	2
B.P. ,, oxidum	$\frac{1}{2}$	2	B.P. Creosotum	1	3
B.P. Arsenii iodidum	$\frac{1}{30}$	—	B.P. Cupri sulphas (tonic, etc.)	$\frac{1}{4}$	2
B.P. Atropina *	$\frac{1}{120}$	$\frac{1}{60}$	B.P. ,, ,, (emetic)	5	10
B.P. Atropinæ sulphas *	$\frac{1}{100}$	$\frac{1}{20}$	Curara	$\frac{1}{30}$	$\frac{1}{4}$
B.P. Belladonnæ radix *	1	5	B.P. Digitalis folia	$\frac{1}{2}$	$1\frac{1}{2}$
B.P. Bismuthi oxidum	5	15	Digitalinum	$\frac{1}{60}$	$\frac{1}{30}$
B.P. ,, carbonas	5	20	B.P. Elaterium	$\frac{1}{24}$	$\frac{1}{8}$
B.P. ,, subnitras	5	20	B.P. Elaterinum	$\frac{1}{40}$	$\frac{1}{10}$
Brucina	$\frac{1}{12}$	$\frac{1}{2}$	Emetina (emetic)	$\frac{1}{4}$	$\frac{1}{2}$
B.P. Butyl-chloral hydras	5	15	B.P. Ergota	20	30
B.P. Caffeina	$\frac{1}{4}$	5	B.P. Ergotin	2	5
B.P. ,, citrate	2	10	Ergotinine (alkaloid)	$\frac{1}{100}$	—
			Euonymin	$\frac{1}{2}$	5
			B.P. Extractum aconiti	$\frac{1}{4}$	1

Solids by Weight; Fluids by Measure	Grains or Minims		Solids by Weight; Fluids by Measure	Grains or Minims	
Extractum aconiti radicis .	$\frac{1}{10}$	$\frac{1}{3}$	B.P. Liquor hydrarg. perchl. . .	30	120
B.P. ,, aloes Barb. . .	2	6	B.P. ,, morph. acet. . . .	10	60
B.P. ,, ,, Socot. . .	2	6	B.P. ,, ,, bimecon. . .	5	40
B.P. ,, belladonnæ . .	$\frac{1}{4}$	1	B.P. ,, ,, hydrochl. . .	10	60
B.P. ,, ,, alcoholic. .	$\frac{1}{10}$	$\frac{1}{4}$	,, opii seda. Battley. .	5	20
B.P. ,, cannabis ind. .	$\frac{1}{4}$	1	B.P. ,, potassæ	15	60
B.P. ,, colchici . . .	$\frac{1}{2}$	2	B.P. ,, potassii permanganatis	2	4
B.P. ,, ,, acet. .	$\frac{1}{2}$	2	B.P. ,, sodæ *	15	60
,, colocynthidis .	5	20	B.P. ,, ,, chlorinatæ . .	10	20
B.P. ,, ,, co.	3	10	B.P. ,, sodii arseniatis . . .	5	10
B.P. ,, conii	2	6	B.P. ,, strychninæ hydrochl.	5	10
U.S.P. ,, digitalis . . .	$\frac{1}{8}$	$\frac{1}{2}$	B.P. Lithii carbonas	3	6
B.P. ,, ergotæ liquid. .	10	30	B.P. ,, citras	5	10
B.P. ,, gelsemii alcohol-icum	$\frac{1}{2}$	2	B.P. Lupulinum	2	5
			B.P. Manganesii oxidum nigrum	4	30
B.P. ,, hyoscyami . .	5	10	B.P. Menthol	$\frac{1}{2}$	2
B.P. ,, jaborandi . .	2	10	Morphina	$\frac{1}{10}$	$\frac{1}{2}$
B.P. ,, jalapæ . . .	5	15	B.P. Morphinæ acetas	$\frac{1}{4}$	$\frac{1}{2}$
B.P. ,, lactucæ . . .	5	15	B.P. ,, hydrochlor. . .	$\frac{1}{4}$	$\frac{1}{2}$
B.P. ,, nucis vomicæ .	$\frac{1}{4}$	1	B.P. ,, sulphas	$\frac{1}{2}$	$\frac{1}{2}$
B.P. ,, opii	$\frac{1}{2}$	2	B.P. Moschus	5	10
B.P. ,, ,, liquidum	10	40	Muscarinæ nitras	$\frac{1}{2}$	$\frac{3}{4}$
B.P. ,, papaveris .	2	5	Narceina	$\frac{1}{4}$	2
B.P. ,, physostigmatis .	$\frac{1}{16}$	$\frac{1}{4}$	Narcotina	1	3
B.P. ,, stramonii . . .	$\frac{1}{4}$	$\frac{1}{2}$	Nicotina	$\frac{1}{8}$	1
B.P. Ferri arsenias	$\frac{1}{16}$	$\frac{1}{8}$	Nitroglycerine	$\frac{1}{100}$	$\frac{1}{30}$
,, et strychninæ citras .	3	8	B.P. ,, tablets (gr. $\frac{1}{100}$)	No. 1	2
,, sulphas exsicc. . . .	1	5	B.P. Nux vomica	1	3
Fuchsine	$\frac{1}{2}$	4	B.P. Oleum crotonis	$\frac{1}{2}$	1
Gelsemina (alkaloid) . . .	$\frac{1}{60}$	$\frac{1}{20}$	B.P. ,, phosphor.	5	10
Homatropine salts. . . .	$\frac{1}{120}$	$\frac{1}{30}$	B.P. ,, sabinæ	1	4
B.P. Hydrargyri iodidum rubrum	$\frac{1}{32}$	$\frac{1}{4}$	B.P. Opium	$\frac{1}{4}$	3
,, ,, viride .	1	3	B.P. Phosphorus *	$\frac{1}{200}$	$\frac{1}{30}$
,, nitras . . .	$\frac{1}{4}$	$\frac{3}{4}$	B.P. Physostigmatis semen * .	1	4
B.P. ,, oxidum rubrum *	$\frac{1}{4}$	1	B.P. Physostigmina *	$\frac{1}{100}$	$\frac{1}{50}$
B.P. ,, perchloridum . .	$\frac{1}{16}$	$\frac{1}{8}$	,, ,, salts . . .	$\frac{1}{60}$	$\frac{1}{30}$
B.P. ,, subchloridum . .	$\frac{1}{2}$	5	B.P. Pilocarpinæ nitras	$\frac{1}{16}$	$\frac{1}{2}$
B.P. Hydrargyrum cum cretâ .	3	8	B.P. Pilula conii co.	5	10
Hyoscyamina	$\frac{1}{120}$	$\frac{1}{40}$	B.P. ,, hydrargyri	3	8
B.P. Injectio apomorphinæ hypo-derm.	2	8	B.P. ,, ,, subchl. co.	5	10
			B.P. ,, phosphori	3	6
B.P. Injectio ergotinæ hypoderm.	3	10	B.P. ,, plumbi c. opio . . .	3	5
B.P. ,, morph. hypoderm.	1	10	B.P. ,, saponis co.	3	5
B.P. Iodoformum	$\frac{1}{2}$	3	Piperina	1	10
B.P. Iodum *	$\frac{1}{4}$	$\frac{1}{2}$	B.P. Plumbi acetas	1	4
B.P. Ipecacuanha (expectorant) .	$\frac{1}{2}$	2	B.P. Potassa sulphurata * . . .	2	8
B.P. ,, (emetic). . .	15	30	Potassii arsenias	$\frac{1}{16}$	$\frac{1}{8}$
Iridin	1	5	,, hypophosph. . . .	1	6
B.P. Jaborandi	5	60	B.P. ,, permangan. . . .	1	5
B.P. Jalapa	10	30	B.P. ,, iodidum	2	20
B.P. Jalapæ resina	2	5	B.P. Pulvis antimonialis . . .	3	5
Lactucarium	3	8	B.P. ,, elaterini co. . . .	$\frac{1}{4}$	5
B.P. Liquor ammoniæ * . . .	10	20	B.P. ,, ipecac. co.	5	15
B.P. ,, arsenicalis . . .	2	8	B.P. ,, kino co.	5	20
B.P. ,, arsen. hydrochl. . .	2	8	B.P. ,, opii co.	2	5
B.P. ,, arsen. et hydrarg. iodid. . . .	10 to 30		Quininæ arsenias	$\frac{1}{4}$	$\frac{1}{2}$
B.P. ,, atropinæ sulph. . .	1	4	B.P. Resina jalapæ	2	5
B.P. ,, bism. et am. citr. . .	30	60	B.P. ,, podophylli	$\frac{1}{4}$	1
B.P. ,, calc. chloridi . . .	15	50	B.P. ,, scammoniæ . . .	3	8
B.P. ,, chlori	10	20	B.P. Sabadilla *	4	6
B.P. ,, Donovani	10	30	B.P. Sabinæ cacumina . . .	4	10
			B.P. Salicinum	3	20

Solids by Weight; Fluids by Measure	Grains or Minims		Solids by Weight; Fluids by Measure	Grains or Minims	
B.P. Santoninum	2	6	B.P. Tinctura digitalis	10	30
B.P. Scammonium	5	10	B.P. ,, ergotæ	5	30
B.P. Scilla	1	3	B.P. ,, gelsemii	5	20
B.P. Sodii arsenias	$\frac{1}{16}$	$\frac{1}{8}$	B.P. ,, hyoscyami	30	60
B.P. ,, hypophosphis	5	10	B.P. ,, iodi	5	20
B.P. ,, iodidum	3	10	B.P. ,, jaborandi	30	60
B.P. ,, sulphocarbolas	10	15	B.P. ,, lobeliæ	10	30
B.P. ,, salicylas	10	30	B.P. ,, æther	10	30
B.P. ,, valerianas	1	5	B.P. ,, nucis vomicæ	10	20
B.P. Strychnina	$\frac{1}{30}$	$\frac{1}{12}$	B.P. ,, opii	5	40
,, salts	$\frac{1}{30}$	$\frac{1}{8}$	B.P. ,, ,, ammon.	30	60
Succus aconiti	10	20	B.P. ,, sabinæ	20	60
B.P. ,, belladonnæ	5	15	,, stramon.	10	30
B.P. ,, conii	30	60	B.P. ,, veratri viridis	5	20
B.P. ,, hyoscyami	30	60	Trimethylaminæ hydro-		
B.P. Syrupus chloral.	30	120	chloras.	2	3
B.P. ,, papaveris	30	60	B.P. Veratrina *	$\frac{1}{16}$	$\frac{1}{10}$
B.P. ,, scillæ	30	60	B.P. Vinum antimonii	5	60
Thallini sulphas	3	8	B.P. ,, colchici	10	30
B.P. Tinctura aconiti	5	15	,, ,, sem.	10	20
,, ,, Fleming	1	2	B.P. ,, ipecac. (emetic)	60	360
B.P. ,, belladonnæ	5	20	B.P. ,, ,, (expectorant)	5	40
B.P. ,, camph. co.	15	60	B.P. ,, opii	10	40
B.P. ,, cannab. ind.	5	20	B.P. Zinci acetas (tonic)	1	2
B.P. ,, capsici	10	20	B.P. ,, ,, (emetic)	10	20
B.P. ,, cantharidis	5	20	B.P. ,, oxidum	2	10
B.P. ,, chloroform et mor-			,, phosphidum	$\frac{1}{16}$	$\frac{1}{8}$
phinæ	5	10	B.P. ,, sulphas (tonic)	1	3
B.P. ,, cimicifugæ	15	60	B.P. ,, ,, (emetic)	10	30
B.P. ,, colchic. sem.	10	30	B.P. ,, valerianas	1	3
B.P. ,, conii	20	60			

The maximum doses in the foregoing table may be regarded as the safe dose
to give; but there are many drugs which have a powerful effect on some
individuals, and others which have quite the opposite. Doses much in
excess of the maxima are sometimes met with; e.g. 10 and 15 grain doses
of calomel in cases of apoplexy, 2-grain doses of extract of Indian hemp
in cases of tetanus. Doses are also given in the chapter on New Remedies.

INDEX.

T

PRINTED BY
SPOTTISWOODE AND CO., NEW-STREET SQUARE
LONDON

AIDS TO DISPENSING.

MODERN PHARMACY has developed many aids to dispensing which have saved the chemist an infinite amount of profitless labour, by supplying him with better products at less cost than he could prepare them without the facilities afforded by the largest laboratories and the greatest amount of special skill.

Such products, manufactured in a large way, possess a greater accuracy than would be possible in the compounding of ordinary prescriptions, and their employment is a great convenience to the physician and chemist, while at the same time the patient receives the required remedy in a superior form.

By this means the patient is often enabled to take medicines and nourishment which in the ordinary way are rejected and thrown away after the first dose or portion, while the use of the more eligible form is continued during the entire time for which it is prescribed.

In dispensing any of such articles, if the prescriber has given any directions the chemist will of course attach them in the usual way, either leaving the original label on or removing it (which is, perhaps, the best way) according to his discretion.

If no directions are given it is naturally inferred that the physician wishes the article used according to the printed directions.

Of the various productions which thus contribute both to the benefit of the patient, the convenience of the physician, and the increased business and profit of the chemist, the following are, perhaps, worthy of special consideration.

EXTRACT OF MALT.

The nutritious, digestive, and vitalising properties of barley malt have been well known for a long time, and the extract has been found the most convenient and efficacious form for use; but it is only in recent years that a perfectly satisfactory preparation has been produced, in which the diastase and other valuable properties of the grain are preserved by the Kepler process, which yields a most elegant and agreeable extract. While it is very useful as a digestive, reconstructive, and vitalising agent, it possesses great utility as a substitute for cod-liver oil, for which it is also a solvent.

It is thus a considerable addition to a chemist's sales and profits, as so many who require cod-liver oil are unable either to take or digest it in its clear state, but who take the extract of malt or the solution of cod-liver oil in extract of malt with relish and benefit.

BEEF AND IRON WINE (FREED FROM TANNIN).

The class of patients for whom physicians so frequently require to prescribe a tonic stimulant are so delicate and sensitive as to the taste of nutriment or tonic that it becomes a matter of much importance that the prescription be as elegant and agreeable as is consistent with utility. Our Beef and Iron Wine takes the place of home-made beef-tea and the old-fashioned solution of iron rust in wine. Such disagreeable mixtures are now, happily for the patient and chemist also, superseded by the elegant and palatable stimulant and blood-food Beef and Iron Wine (Burroughs), which has given such general satisfaction to the medical profession and increased the business and profits of the trade.

The "Tabloid" form of medication has greatly increased the use of the drugs so compressed by rendering them at once more agreeable and effective.

TABLOIDS OF COMPRESSED DRUGS.

Drugs intended for local effect upon the mouth and throat are compressed very hard and dissolve slowly, producing the effect of a concentrated and continuous gargle. One of the tabloids placed in the mouth at night will be barely dissolved before morning, and the form renders them easily retained while speaking or singing.

For internal administration they are very desirable, as their shape is nearest the form of the throat, so that they are more easily swallowed than any other form of pill. Drugs which are intended to be swallowed are compressed lightly (as Quinine, dry Cascara Extract, Antipyrin, and the Tabloid Triturates) are quite porous, and very soluble. This can be readily observed either by the constitutional effect or by simply suspending one of the above tabloids in water, when they will be observed to disintegrate immediately and to dissolve in less time than any ordinary hand or machine made pill.

As many invalids will take drugs in this form who refuse the ordinary methods of administration, the drugs being made more available and useful their employment is considerably increased.

HYPODERMIC "TABLOIDS."

The serious disadvantages attending the employment of ordinary solutions for hypodermic medication have considerably hindered this method of use, but all objections are now apparently removed by the preparation of the soluble hypodermic tabloids in which the alkaloids are supplied in a permanent and soluble form in accurately divided doses.

"LANOLINE" LIEBREICH.

To Professor Liebreich is due the credit of discovering that wool-fat is much more readily absorbed by the skin and hair than ordinary fat or petroleum derivatives. This might reasonably be expected, as such fat is natural to these tissues.

The introduction of "Lanoline," by increasing the activity of medicaments used with it in ointments, makes them more widely useful. Its effect upon the skin is peculiarly soothing and healing, restoring its natural functions, elasticity, and texture. It does not, like vaseline, remain like a varnish upon the skin, but is quickly and with a little friction completely absorbed, carrying the medicament, if any, with it.

"Lanoline" is naturally the best basis for cold cream, pomade, and soap, as by the use of such toilet preparations the skin and hair are preserved in a natural condition. Lanoline Pomade is now prepared with the addition of naphthol, and in this combination is found most effective in removing dandruff and scaly affections of the scalp.

VALOID FLUID EXTRACTS.

These exact and elegant fluid extracts are of the greatest service as aids to dispensing, for, by their use, tinctures, syrups, infusions, decoctions, &c., can be prepared immediately by simple dilution with the proper menstruum.

The Valoid Fluid Extracts are prepared from fresh drugs of standard quality and carefully assayed wherever practicable, a uniform product is secured, representing the full value of the alkaloid, resinoid, or other active principles. They are the most eligible of all standardised preparations.

PHARMACEUTICAL APPARATUS.

Tincture-presses and drug-mills are also valuable aids to the dispenser. A good pharmaceutical still is also sometimes desirable.

Burroughs, Wellcome & Co., of Snow Hill Buildings, London, E.C., call attention to their drug-mills and screw-presses, as per illustration in *The Chemists' and Druggists' Diary*, which have been before the trade for several years, and are considered the most practically useful and easily managed of any, while the Remington Still possesses the important advantage of having a condenser composed of several straight tubes, which can be easily cleaned, and of being readily improvised into an evaporating-dish or water-bath.

Burroughs, Wellcome & Co. also ask particular attention to the Zyminised or Peptonised Suppositories, which are prepared either with milk or meat, and which are of the greatest utility in rectal feeding, when for any reason it is inadmissible to take food by the mouth.

They will be happy to furnish particulars upon request to any chemist of these and any other new pharmaceutical products or apparatus which they introduce.

"Tabloids" and "Tablets"—*continued.*

Livingstone's Rousers. Dose, 2 or 3 in malarial fevers.

Manganese Dioxide, 2 gr., 25 in bot. 8/6 doz. 100 in bot. 32/ doz. Dose, 1 to 5.

Nitro-Glycerine (Trinitrine), 1-100 and 1-50 **gr.** 25 in oval bot. 7/6 doz. ; 100 in bot. 18/ doz; Dose, 1.

Papain, 2 gr. each, in bots. of 100.

Pepsin Pure, 1 gr., 25 in oval bot. 14/ doz. ; 100 in bot. 42/ doz. Dose, 1 to 5.

Pepsin Saccharated, 5 gr., 100 in bot. 32/ doz. Dose, 1 to 3.

Peptonic, 25 in oval bot. 14/ doz. ; 100 in bot. 48/ doz. Dose, 1 or 2 after meals.

Phenacetin, 5 gr., 25 in oval bot. 24/ doz. ; 100 in bot. 72/ doz. Dose, 1 to 3 every four hours.

Potash Bicarb., 5 gr. 25 in oval bot. 4/6 doz. ; 100 in bot. 12/6 doz. Dose, 1 to 4.

Potash Chlorate, 5 gr., 30 in box, 4/ ; 30 in oval bot. 4/6 doz. ; 100 in box or bot. 8/6 doz. Dose, 1 slowly dissolved in the mouth.

Potash Chlorate with Borax, 30 in box, 4/ doz. ; 30 in oval bot. 4/6 doz. ; 100 in box or bot. 8/6 doz. Dose, 1 slowly dissolved in the mouth.

Potash Nitrate (*Sal Prunella*), 100 in bot. 14/ doz. Dose, 1 slowly dissolved in the mouth.

Potash Permanganate, 1 gr , 100 in bot. 18/ doz. ; 2 gr., 100 in bot. 32/ doz. Dose, 1 or 2.

Potassium Bromide, 5 gr., 100 in bot. 18/ doz. ; 10 gr., 100 in bot. 32/ doz. Dose, 1 or 2.

Potassium Iodide, 5 gr., 100 in bot. 36/ doz. Dose, 1 or more with meals.

Quinine Bisulphate (soluble), ½ gr., 50 in oval bot. 8/ doz. ; 100 in bot. 12/ doz. ; 1 gr., 36 in oval bot. 8/ doz. ; 100 in bot. 15/ doz. ; 2 gr., 24 in oval bot. 8/ doz. ; 100 in bot. 24/ doz. ; 3 gr., 24 in oval bot. 12/ doz. ; 100 in bot. 35/ doz. ; 5 gr., 24 in oval bot. 17/6 doz. ; 100 in bot. 50/ doz.

Quin. Bisulph., 1 gr.
Iron Hypophos., 2 gr. ⎫ Dose, 1 thrice daily
Arsenic, 1/50 gr.   ⎬ after meals, swallowed
Strych. Sulph., 1/50 gr. ⎪ or previously dissolved
Saccharin, 1/100 gr.   ⎭ in water.

Rhubarb Comp., B.P., 3 gr.. 24 in oval bot. 7/6 doz. ; 100 in bot. 22/ doz. Dose, 1 to 5.

Rhubarb and Magnesia, 5 gr., 24 in oval bot. 7/6 doz. ; 100 in bot. 22/ doz. Dose, 1 to 5

Rhubarb and Soda, 5 gr., 24 in oval bot. 7/6 doz. ; 100 in bot. 22/ doz. Dose, 1 to 5.

Rhubarb, 3 gr., 24 in oval bot. 7/6 doz. ; 100 in bot. 22/ doz. Dose, 2 to 4.

Saccharin, ½ gr., 25 in tube, /6, 4/ doz. ; 60 in tube, 1/, 8/ doz. ; in oval bot. of 200, 2/6, 24/ doz. These contain 90 per cent. of Pure Saccharin. Substitute for sugar in diabetes.

Salol, 5 gr., 100 in bot. 48/ doz. Dose, 1 or 2.

Soda Bicarbonate, 5 gr., 30 in oval bot. 4/6 doz. ; 100 in bot., 12/6 doz. Dose, 1 to 6.

Soda Chlorate, 5 gr.. 100 in bot. 22/ doz. Dose, 1 to lowly dissolved in the mouth.

Soda Chlorate and Borax, 5 gr., 25 in oval bot. 7/6 doz. ; 100 in bot. 18/ doz. Dose, 1 to 4, slowly dissolved in the mouth.

Soda-Mint ("or *Neutralising Tabloid*", 25 in oval bot. 7/6 doz. ; 100 in bot, 18/ doz. Dose, 1 to 4.

Soda Salicylate, 3 gr., 100 in bot. 28/ doz. ; 5 gr., 100 in bot. 38/ doz. Dose, 1 to 4.

Soda Sulpho-carbolate, 5 gr., 100 in bot. 28/ doz. Dose, 1 to 3.

"Tabloids" and "Tablets"—*continued.*

Sodium Bromide, 5 gr., 100 in bot, 18/ doz. ; 10 gr. 100 in bot. 32/ doz. Dose, 2 to 4.

Sodium Iodide, 5 gr., 100 in bot. 48/ doz. Dose, 1 or more, with meals.

Sodium Taurocholas (coated with Keratin), 4 gr., 100 in bot. Dose, 1 three times a day.

Strophanthus (2 minims of Tincture in each), 50 in oval bot. 8/6 doz. ; 100 in bot. 16/ doz.

Sulphonal, 5 grs., 25 in bot. 30/ doz. ; 100 in bot. 96/ doz. Dose, 1 to 4.

Tannin, 2½ gr., 100 in bot. 22/ doz. Dose, 1 or more as a styptic.

Test Tabloids (for preparing Fehling's Solution). Portable and convenient Test for Sugar, 18/ doz.

"Thirst Tabloids." (Contain Citric Acid, &c.), 8/ doz.

Tonic Comp. ⎧ Iron Pyrophos., 2 gr. ⎫ Dose, 1
            ⎨ Quinine, 1 gr.   ⎬ with
            ⎩ Strychnine, 1/100 gr. ⎭ meals.
25 in oval bot. 12/6 doz. ; 100 in bot. 36/ doz.

Trinitrine (*Nitro-Glycerine*), 1/100 gr. and 1/50 gr., 25 in oval bot. 7/6 doz. ; 100 in bot. 18/ doz. Dose, 1.

Trinitrine and Amyl Nitrite, 25 in oval bot. 12/ doz. ; 100 in bot. 36/ doz. Dose, 1.

Trinitrine Comp. ⎧ Trinitrine, 1/100 gr.   ⎫
                 ⎪ Nitrite of Amyl, ¼ gr. ⎬ Dose,
                 ⎨ Capsicum, 1/50 gr.   ⎪ 1.
                 ⎩ Menthol, 1/50 gr.   ⎭
25 in oval bot, 12/6 doz. ; 100 in bot. 36/ doz.

Urethane, 5 gr., 25 in bot. 16/ doz. ; 100 in bot. 40/ doz. Dose, 1 to 4.

Voice (Potash, Borax, and Cocaine), 30 in box, 8/ doz. ; in bot. 8/6 doz. ; 80 in box, 16/ doz. Dose, 1 slowly dissolved on the tongue.

Warburg's Tincture (½ drachm in each).

Zinc Sulphate, 1 gr., 100 in bot. 18/ doz.

Zinc Sulpho-Carbolate, 2 gr., 100 in bot. 18/ doz.

Zymine (3 gr. Ext. Pancreatis), 25 in bot. 18/ doz. ; 100 in bot., 48/ doz.

Zymine Comp. (Ext. Pancreatis, 2 gr. ; Ipecac., 1-10 gr. ; and Bismuth Subnitrate, 3 gr.), 25 in bot. 18/ doz. ; 100 in bot. 48/ doz.

"Tabloids" of Triturated Drugs.

(Prepared by Burroughs, Wellcome & Co.)

In bottles of 100, 8/6 doz., and tubes of 25, 4/6 doz.

Aconite Tinct., 1 min.
Arsenious Acid, 1/100 gr. **and** 1/50 gr.
Belladonna Tinct., 1 min.
Calcium Sulphide, 1/10 gr.
Capsicum Tinct., 1 min.
Digitalis Tinct., 1 min.
Hydrarg. Perchlor., 1/100 gr.
Hydrarg. cum Cretâ (Grey Powder), 1/3 gr.
Hydrarg. Subchlor. (Calomel), 1/10 gr.
Hyoscyamus Tinct., 1 min.
Nux Vomica Tinct., 1 min.
Tinct. Camph. Co. (Paregoric), 2 min.

In bottles of 50 and tubes of 25—

Anti-Constipation ⎧ Aloin, 1/5 gr.
                  ⎪ Belladonna Ext., 1/8 gr.
                  ⎨ Strych., 1/60 gr.
                  ⎩ Ipecac., 1/16 gr.

Apomorphine Muriate, 1/50 gr.
Atropine Sulph., 1/100 gr.
Digitalin, 1/100 gr.
Euonymin Resin, 1/8 gr.
Hydrarg. Iod. Rub., 1/20 gr.

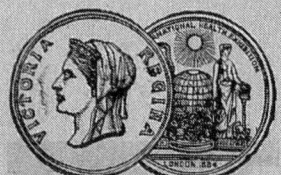

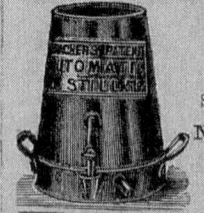

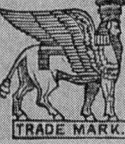

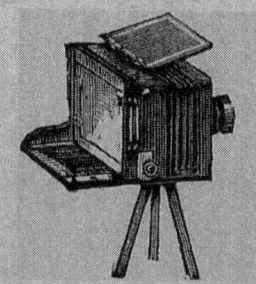 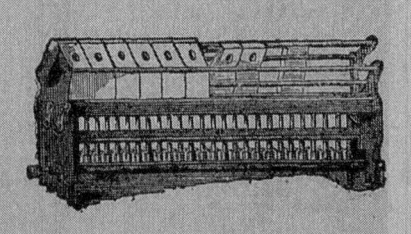

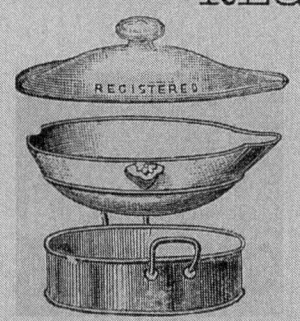

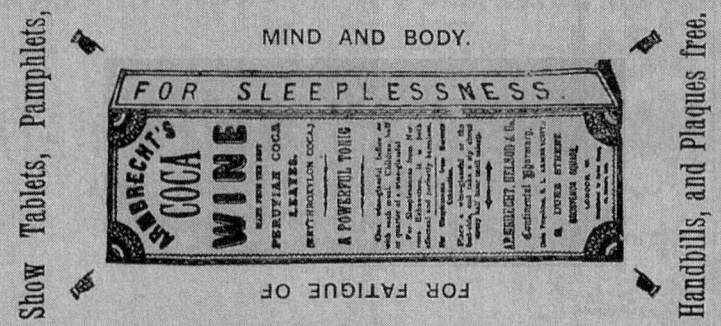

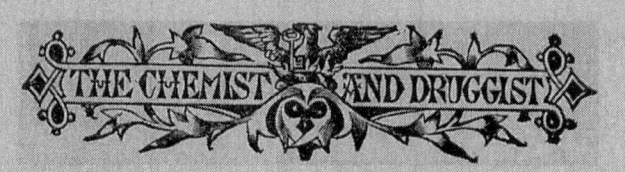

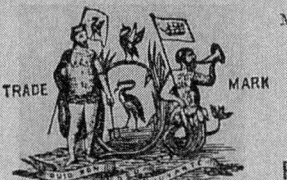
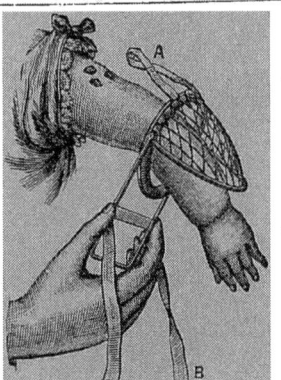
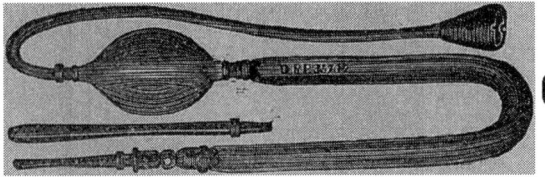

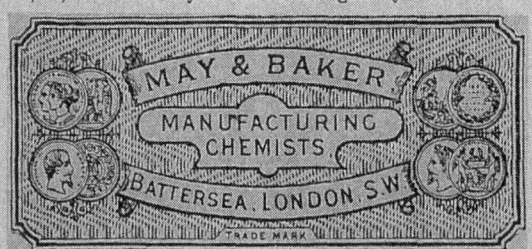

CPSIA information can be obtained
at www.ICGtesting.com
Printed in the USA
LVHW040846181222
735461LV00004B/125